RELAX
SLEEP
THRIVE

Your 5-Week Journey to Peaceful, Restorative Sleep

By Amanda Chocko, NTP

I would like to dedicate this book to the women who are fed up with sleepless nights.

To those who have tossed and turned, counted countless sheep, and searched for solace in the darkness.
This book is for you, the resilient souls who yearn for restorative slumber and the energy to face each new day with vitality.

May the wisdom within these pages illuminate your path to peaceful sleep, and may you find the rest you deserve.

For permission requests, email to the publisher via the website below.

First Edition, Softcover

Published by Amanda Chocko

www.AmandaChocko.com
ISBN: 979-8-9887549-0-9

Cover Design by Rivka Hodgkinson
Interior Design by Rivka Hodgkinson

Printed in the United States

IMPORTANT NOTE

The information presented in this book is intended for educational and informational purposes only. It is not a substitute for professional medical advice, diagnosis, or treatment. Always seek the advice of your physician or another qualified health provider with any questions you may have regarding a medical condition. Never disregard professional medical advice or delay in seeking it because of something you have read in this book or related materials.

The author and publisher of this book are not medical professionals, and the content provided is not intended to replace or supersede the recommendations of your healthcare provider. Every individual is unique, and what may be suitable for one person may not be suitable for another. Prior to making any significant changes to your health-related habits, including changes related to sleep, nutrition, supplements, or medications, consult with a qualified medical professional who can assess your specific needs, provide personalized guidance, and monitor your progress. The author and publisher disclaim any liability for any adverse effects or consequences resulting from the use or application of the information contained in this book.

TABLE OF CONTENTS

INTRODUCTION

Unraveling the Insomnia Conundrum

Here begins the first day of your quest for peaceful, restorative sleep.

Does the following sound familiar? After a day crammed full of errands, work, and life's little dramas, all you crave is the sanctuary of your comfy bed. You switch off the lights, snuggle under the covers, and ... boom! It's like someone flicked the 'on' switch in your brain. Or, worse yet, you plunge into the depths of sleep only to be rocketed awake at the ungodly hour of 3 a.m., thoughts whirring like a relentless spinning wheel.

I've had my fair share of sleepless nights and midnight-stress parties. I have tried it all while trying to get a good night's sleep. Things such as various 'bedtime brews,' like the classic Sleepy Time tea. Sure, it got me off to dreamland, but then there were the oh-so-frequent nocturnal bathroom visits. I've also tried unwinding with a nice glass of wine, which worked a charm... until that unfriendly 3 a.m. wake-up call, leaving me wrestling with sleep yet again.

My pursuit of a restful night's sleep saw me dabbling with all kinds of 'quick fixes,' but it wasn't until I was grappling with the bear that is chronic insomnia that I knew it was time to dig deeper. I embarked on a journey to uncover the secrets of slumber, peeling back the layers to expose the root causes of my sleep disruptions.

Fast-forward two years and a transformation from an insomniac to a self-proclaimed "sleep detective," I'm pleased to say I've mastered the art of a peaceful night's rest. I still have the occasional restless night, but I can typically connect the dots and quickly steer my sleep back on course.

I want to save you the many sleepless nights and failed attempts. Now, I'm going to show you step by step what works for you. Join me as I share the wealth of knowledge and experience I've gained along my own journey. I'm excited to guide you towards taking back control of your sleep, empowering you to wake up refreshed, rejuvenated, and ready to seize the day - every day!

About This Book

Welcome to Relax, Sleep, Thrive: Your 5-week Journey to Peaceful, Restorative Sleep! If you're holding this book, chances are sleepless nights have been stealing your zest for life. It's time for that to change.

As a Nutritional Therapy Practitioner and Sleep Coach, I wrote Relax, Sleep, Thrive as more than a book. It is a comprehensive 5-week journey toward conquering insomnia and reclaiming rejuvenating sleep. It is a program specially designed to help you unravel the root causes of your sleep struggles and equip you with actionable strategies to implement healthy sleep patterns.

Think of this book as your interactive guide, your personal sleep coach that you can access any time of the day or night. It's not just a book to read; it's a workbook for you to engage with, reflect on, and learn from. Packed with journaling activities and exercises, it's designed for you to write in it, scribble notes, highlight important points, and make it truly your own. The more you interact, the more insights you'll gain into your unique sleep patterns.

Each week includes a blend of enlightening content and practical action items tailored to transform your sleep habits.

Week One: Laying the Foundation

This week is about setting the stage for your sleep journey. Restful sleep relies on a solid base like a house needs a strong foundation. We'll explore the mechanics of sleep and its crucial role in your health and start shaping your sleep hygiene.

Week Two: Become a Sleep Detective

It's time to connect the dots. You'll uncover the everyday habits that may sabotage your sleep and learn how to tweak your day for a restful night. By identifying and adjusting these patterns, you'll empower yourself to take charge of your sleep destiny.

Week Three: Mastering Mind Management

Get set to uncover the secret to managing the anxiety, stress, and relentless mind chatter that keeps you up at night. You will be equipped with tools and techniques to help you drift off to dreamland.

Week Four: Your Sleep Toolbox

Dive into the world of sleep helpers this week. From apps to weighted blankets, you'll fill your sleep toolbox with an array of sleep-enhancing tools to personalize and optimize your sleep experience.

Week Five: Digging Deeper

As we progress your sleep journey, this week is dedicated to troubleshooting persistent issues and discussing the next steps in your personalized sleep journey. We'll explore advanced strategies and tools, ensuring you have a comprehensive approach to conquering even the trickiest sleep challenges.

How to Use This Book

I suggest progressing through the program day by day. This approach lets you thoroughly digest the material without feeling overwhelmed. And while it's essential to stay committed, remember that occasional setbacks are natural. Strive for progress, not perfection.

Once you get to the end, you will find additional resources that you can use to continue your journey beyond the first five weeks. Peaceful, restorative sleep is a life-long journey, and you are worth it!

WEEK 1

Laying the Foundation

Week One is where the groundwork for your sleep transformation is laid. We'll delve into the inner workings of sleep and its fundamental impact on your well-being. You will set the foundations of sleep hygiene by establishing a consistent sleep schedule, cultivating a serene sleep environment, crafting a soothing bedtime routine, and monitoring your sleep patterns.

As you incorporate these healthy sleep habits into your life, you'll be well on your way to rejuvenating rest.

Let's embark on this empowering journey towards revitalizing your sleep!

DAY 1

Your Baseline Sleep Assessment

Think of this as your personal 'sleep snapshot,' capturing all the details of your current sleep patterns. This invaluable tool will give you a clear starting point and a concrete way to measure your progress throughout the program.

From sleep duration to wake-up times, this assessment dives deep into the various aspects of your sleep. It may even shine a light on specific patterns or habits you weren't previously aware of. By understanding where you're starting from, you can better tailor the program to your needs and monitor how much you've improved by the end.

Don't worry if your sleep habits are far from perfect - that's why you're here! And remember, honesty is key. The more accurate you are, the better we can help you transform your nights.

At the end of our journey together, you'll revisit this assessment. By then, you'll be amazed at how far you've come! So, let's get started with this exciting first step towards reclaiming your nights. After all, understanding is the first step to improvement.

Sleep Assessment

This sleep assessment reveals the extent of your sleep problems.
Rate each symptom according to the scale below.

Point Scale:

(0) never (1) 1-2 days/week (2) 3- 4 days/week (3) 5-7 days/week

_____ I need alcohol or medications to relax before bed.

_____ I have trouble falling asleep

_____ I cannot fall asleep because I am worrying about things

_____ I wake up more than once during the night

_____ I toss and turn at night

_____ I wake up and need to go to the bathroom

_____ I wake up before my alarm and cannot fall back asleep

_____ I have trouble waking up

_____ I need caffeine in the morning to get me going

_____ I have trouble concentrating during the day

_____ I have night sweats

_____ I wake up suddenly with a strong sense of anxiety

_____ I have difficulty falling asleep because of chronic pain

_____ I am sleepy during the day

_____ I find myself irritable or unable to tolerate normal stress

_____ I often have a hard time remembering things

_____ I doze off during the day while working and/or driving

_____ I often feel like I am in a daze or brain fog

_____ **Total Score**   9

DAY 2

The Ripple Effects of Restless Nights

Let's get real - securing sound sleep is nothing less than striking gold for your overall health and well-being. I often compare a sleepless night to building a house of cards - a single jittery moment, and the entire structure tumbles. Just one bad night can lay waste to your motivation, focus, memory, mood, energy, willpower, resilience, productivity, and even your decisions around exercise and food.

Our society is grappling with a chronic issue of sleep deprivation. The National Sleep Foundation has estimated that at least 30% of us are wrestling with some form of sleep disruption. For some, it's the struggle of falling asleep; for others, it's the frustrating pattern of waking in the wee hours, unable to drift back into dreamland. Then there are those who just can't score high-quality sleep. The repercussions of poor sleep extend far beyond daily function and can snowball into a host of health problems.

If you're joining me on this journey, I'm confident you're all too aware of the grim toll insomnia is taking on your life. But to add some fuel to your commitment, let's delve into the impacts of this wellness-stealer in a bit more detail.

Short-term Fallout of Sleep Deprivation

Even a single restless night can ripple into your day, and its consequences are more profound than you might think. Just a brief encounter with sleep deprivation can:

- Sap your energy and make the thought of exercising feel as daunting as climbing Mount Everest.
- Throw your emotional balance off-kilter, making mood swings and irritability your unwanted companions.
- Cloud your mind, compromising concentration and making decisions feel like navigating a maze.
- Undermine your productivity, placing your goals on distant horizons that seem harder to reach.
- Diminish your alertness, raising the stakes for potential mishaps, whether you're on the road or at your desk.

Poor sleep will also mess with your hunger hormones and metabolism. Let's take a closer look.

Feeling Hangry?

Ever found yourself feeling peckish following a night of restless sleep? I've often noticed an uptick in snacking and cravings throughout the day when my sleep is compromised. Poor sleep can substantially skew the hunger hormones - leptin and ghrelin - which are instrumental in managing appetite and energy balance in the body.

Sleep deprivation leads to a drop in leptin, a hormone that signals when you've had enough to eat. This results in increased hunger and a diminished sense of fullness. Conversely, lack of sleep can boost ghrelin levels - the hormone that turns your appetite dial-up, making you susceptible to high-calorie, high-fat food temptations.

Sleepless nights have also been associated with impaired glucose metabolism and insulin sensitivity, adding to the problems of increased hunger and reduced satiety. Plus, sleep deprivation can mess with your brain's decision-making abilities and impulse control, making it harder to resist less healthy food choices and maintain portion control.

Sleep is more than a simple recharge; it's essential for navigating life's daily challenges with grace and efficiency. Now let's explore the long-term consequences of insomnia.

Long-term Repercussions

When insomnia becomes a frequent visitor, it doesn't just leave you with a groggy morning. Its lingering presence can snowball into severe health issues.

Consider the following repercussions of chronic insomnia:

- Chronic insomnia can be a gateway to devastating health challenges, including heart disease, diabetes, and obesity.
- Your emotional well-being becomes fragile, making room for mood disorders like depression and anxiety.
- Essential cognitive functions, such as memory, attention, and executive decision-making, start deteriorating.
- Recent studies draw a worrying connection between chronic insomnia and neurological ailments like Parkinson's, Alzheimer's, and dementia.
- Older adults with persistent insomnia face an elevated risk of mortality.
- What's worse, a self-perpetuating cycle can form where the mere fear of insomnia aggravates its intensity.

As you can see, the implications of insomnia are far-reaching. Don't fret if you are currently feeling these impacts. You are well on your way to conquering your insomnia once and for all. But it is going to take commitment, which leads us to today's action item.

Action Item: The Sleep Oath

It's time to gear up and commit to taking back your sleep! Sleep recovery isn't a leisurely walk in the park but rather a marathon requiring commitment, resolve, and an unwavering spirit. It might mean reshaping your daily patterns, adopting fresh habits, and bidding farewell to some of your cozy routines (yes, we're looking at you, midnight Netflix marathons). This may send ripples through your relationships and social calendars. Without a full-hearted commitment, you may find this program is like pedaling a bicycle with flat tires—you exert effort but make little progress.

Your Pledge to Nightly Serenity

I, _____, hereby make my sleep restoration a towering priority.

I pledge to:

1. Forge my sleep into an unyielding, non-negotiable pillar of my daily life.

2. Proclaim my commitment to the world, or at least to those who might be impacted.

3. Tread the path of optimal sleep hygiene, even if it takes me to unfamiliar territories.

4. Weed out habits that might pose as sleep thieves.

5. Chronicle my journey with a keen eye, unmasking the true culprits of my sleep issues.

6. Try, test, and tweak potential solutions, embracing the spirit of experimentation.

7. Conquer my sleep challenges, emerging victorious within the next 30 days.

What is Your Why?

Now that you have taken your oath, it is equally important to know your "Why." Why is it important for you to fix your sleep? How will your life be better as a result? What is at stake if you don't make a change?

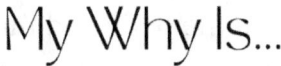

My Why Is...

When you feel yourself slipping back into the habits that are detrimental to your sleep, always revisit your "Why." Remind yourself of your pledge. Now rest up. Tomorrow, we delve into the mechanics of sleep!

DAY 3

Sync Your Rhythms

Kudos for conquering your first two days! You've assessed your sleep quality, made your commitment, and you know your "Why." Today, let's delve into the science of sleep and its profound effects on the body and mind.

Knowledge is Power!

So, you're all set on a quest to conquer insomnia and reclaim the good night's sleep you've been missing, right? The first step in this noble pursuit is to get acquainted with the inner workings of sleep itself. When you understand the gears and levers that control our sleep, you'll be well on your way to spotting the connection between your daily lifestyle and those pesky bouts of insomnia. The magic behind a restful night's sleep is spun by two primary actors: circadian rhythms and sleep pressure.

The Circadian Ballet

Imagine circadian rhythms as a 24-hour dance our bodies do, guided by the ebb and flow of light and darkness. This rhythmic performance schedules all the essential processes, like when to release hormones, how our digestion flows, how our blood pressure fluctuates, when we get hungry, and when our mental energy peaks. And, of course, the star players in this dance are the two hormones: melatonin and cortisol.

Melatonin, the lullaby that our pineal gland sings, signals that it's time to wind down and tuck into bed. As the day wanes and night creeps in, our melatonin production goes into overdrive, whispering to our bodies, "It's bedtime." As we sleep, melatonin levels gently decline, making room for its energetic counterpart, cortisol.

Cortisol is our built-in alarm clock, pumped out by our adrenal glands. It's the bugle call that tells our bodies to rise and shine, kick-starting our day with a burst of energy.

In an ideal world, melatonin and cortisol maintain a beautifully choreographed balance. But if cortisol decides to gatecrash the sleep party, it can toss our restful night into chaos.

Sleep Pressure: The Need to Snooze

Circadian rhythms aren't the only game in town. Our bodies also cook up a chemical called adenosine that piles up in our brains throughout the day, acting as our personal sleep countdown. This is called "sleep pressure". The tug-of-war between a rising tide of melatonin and the build-up of adenosine ultimately sends us surrendering to the sweet call of sleep.

As we slumber, adenosine slowly vacates our system, and after about 7 to 8 hours of quality sleep, it's all gone, leaving us refreshed and ready to seize the day. But if we short-change our sleep, this adenosine lingers into the next day, leaving us groggy and out of sorts.

In this journey, we will suss out the culprits that could be riling up your cortisol or messing with your sleep pressure. I'll arm you with the knowledge and tools to tame your sleep and restore it to its rightful rhythm. Speaking of rhythms, it is time for today's action item.

Action Item: Setting Your Sleep Schedule

Let's Get in Sync (not the band, your circadian rhythms)!

Your body is an amazing machine that thrives on regularity, consistency, and rhythm. This includes the ebb and flow of meals, workouts, and, most importantly, your snooze sessions. Being consistent with your sleep times makes all the difference. Yes, even on weekends!

Are you thinking, "Really? What about my Friday night social life? Or my luxurious weekend lie-ins?" Believe it or not, re-establishing your sleep equilibrium will require some sacrifices (remember the sleep oath you took?).

Step one in reclaiming your slumber is setting a consistent wake-up time that allows you to start your day stress-free. For instance, if your wake-up time is 6:00 AM, enjoy the calm of early morning with a leisurely coffee, light exercise, a nourishing breakfast, and a relaxed preparation for the day. I've come to love my peaceful morning time before the rest of the family gets up. Adhering to this schedule will help tune your body clock so that you might eventually ditch the alarm clock once and for all.

Your Sleep Schedule

Jot down your daily wake-up time:

My unwavering wake-up time is _____.

Next up, you need to nail down your bedtime. On average, individuals require 7 to 9 hours of rest to function at their peak. Depending on your personal sleep needs, count backwards from your wake-up time, and allow an extra 15 to 30 minutes as a buffer for drifting off to sleep.

Jot down your daily bedtime:

My steadfast bedtime is _____.

Example:
Wake-up time: 6:00 AM
Sleep requirement: 8 hours
Bedtime: 9:30 PM

For those who struggle with sleep-onset insomnia, waiting until you're genuinely sleepy before hitting the sack is crucial. If you climb into bed without feeling tired, your brain might associate your bed with wakefulness rather than sleep, making falling asleep an uphill task. So, if you're not drowsy at bedtime, engage in a relaxing or non-stimulating activity until sleepiness sets in. This could involve reading a book, listening to soothing music, meditating, or journaling. By waiting until you're authentically sleepy to crawl into bed, you increase your chances of falling asleep swiftly and enjoying a restful night. We'll delve deeper into establishing your bedtime routine later in the program. Begin incorporating your sleep schedule tonight.

DAY 4

Sleep Stages - Your Journey Into Dreamland

You're now well on your way to becoming a sleep guru, armed with the know-how of why sleep is such a big deal for our overall well-being and the dual forces that drive it: circadian rhythms and sleep pressure. Today we'll explore the ebb and flow of sleep stages and their significant role in your quest for restorative sleep.

Quantity vs. Quality

You might think, "All I want is to snooze through the night. Is that too much to ask?" Of course, uninterrupted sleep is a worthy goal, but there's more to the story: the quality of your sleep.

Just as a gourmet meal is about more than filling your stomach, quality sleep nourishes your body and mind uniquely. The various stages of sleep, light sleep, deep sleep, and REM sleep, each have their unique roles in reviving our bodies and minds.

Balancing these stages is the secret sauce to waking up rejuvenated, ready to leap into the day. Getting familiar with these stages can empower us to make wise choices that enhance sleep quality, thereby boosting our mood, sharpening our focus, and bolstering our overall health. Let's sneak a peek into these stages.

21

The 4 Stages of Sleep

Stage 1 - The Prelude to Slumber: This is when drowsiness sets in, and your body gears up for a restful night. Muscles start to relax (sometimes twitching a bit) as you gradually detach from your surroundings.

Stage 2 - Light Sleep: Your breathing finds its rhythm, your heart rate takes it down a notch, and your body temperature starts to dip as you enter light sleep.

Stage 3 & 4 - Deep Sleep: The ultimate restoration stage. Here, your heart and breathing find their zen, muscles let go, and it's a tough task to wake you up. Deep sleep is the elixir for muscle growth, repair, and immune system regulation. It's the "body restorative" phase, when your brain sweeps away the day's accumulated toxins.

Stage 5 - REM Sleep: This is your mind's spa time. REM sleep refuels cognitive function, consolidates memory, regulates mood, processes emotions, and sparks creativity. The "mental restorative" phase is also where dreams come to life.

Striking a balance between sleep quality and sleep duration is key. Excellent quality sleep can fall short if the duration is consistently too short. Conversely, a long but restless sleep can leave you feeling groggy.

The Golden Ratio of Sleep

What is the golden ratio of sleep? A blend of high-quality slumber spanning an adequate duration, usually between 7 and 9 hours for most adults. This ensures a complete tour of all the essential sleep stages, leaving you recharged and ready to take on the day.

Having demystified sleep, its importance, and its pitfalls, you are ready for today's action item: tracking your sleep.

Action Item: The Morning Sleep Journal

One of the most important steps you can take on your journey to better sleep is to understand your current sleep patterns. Before we start making changes, we need to establish a baseline — a detailed understanding of how you sleep now. That's where the Morning Sleep Journal comes in.

Your Morning Sleep Journal is an essential tool for uncovering the mysteries of your sleep habits. By documenting your sleep and wake times, the ease with which you fall asleep, any nighttime disruptions, and how you feel in the morning, we can begin to understand the patterns and nuances of your sleep.

For today's action item, take a few minutes to fill out your Morning Sleep Journal based on last night's sleep.

Moving forward, you will fill out your Morning Journal as soon as you wake up. This will ensure that your sleep experience is fresh in your mind.

Morning Sleep Journal

Complete this each morning to see the impact on your daily sleep!

Today's Date: _____   Bedtime Last Night: _____

How well did you fall asleep?

___ Easily   ___ It took a while   ___ It was difficult

Describe what it was like falling asleep:

Did you wake up and struggle to fall back asleep?

___ Not at all   ___ Once or twice   ___ Multiple times

Describe your experience:

Wake-Up Time: _____   Total Hours of Sleep _____

How did you feel after waking up?

___ Refreshed   ___ Just okay   ___ Tired

Notes:

DAY 5

Creating Your Sleep Sanctuary

Good morning! How did you sleep last night?

Your bedroom is not just a space where you retire at the end of the day - it's your personal sanctuary, your escape into the soothing realm of dreams. It is, therefore, crucial to transform this personal space into a tranquil sleep haven. A relaxing sleep environment encourages your mind to wind down and prepare for a good night's rest.

Today, we'll explore strategies to help you create the optimal sleep environment that ensures sound sleep and improves the overall quality of your rest.

Before we dive into today's topic, be sure to fill out your morning sleep journal on the next page.

Morning Sleep Journal

Complete this each morning to see the impact on your daily sleep!

Today's Date: _____   Bedtime Last Night: _____

How well did you fall asleep?

___ Easily   ____ It took a while   ____ It was difficult

Describe what it was like falling asleep:

Did you wake up and struggle to fall back asleep?

___ Not at all   ____ Once or twice   ____ Multiple times

Describe your experience:

Wake-Up Time: _____   Total Hours of Sleep _____

How did you feel after waking up?

___ Refreshed   ____ Just okay   ____ Tired

Notes:

Establish a No-work/No-screen Zone

Now that you have completed your sleep journal, let's dive into today's topic. For optimal relaxation, it is important that you train your mind to associate your bedroom with rest. Make it a rule that no TV, working, eating, or any other distracting activities are allowed in the bedroom. This means no laptops, tablets, or smartphones. These electronic devices emit blue light, disrupting your sleep by suppressing melatonin production. In addition, they can cause nervous system arousal, further hindering sleep. The bedroom should be reserved for sleeping and intimacy with your partner only.

Tidy Up

Cluttered spaces can create stress and anxiety, and that's not what you want in your bedroom. Remove all clutter from your bedroom to create a peaceful and calming environment. This includes clothes on the floor, piles of books, and any other items that don't belong in the bedroom. Keep your bedroom clean and tidy, and your mind will follow suit.

Keep Your Cool

Even if you are not experiencing night sweats, a comfortable bedroom temperature is vital for sleep quality. According to the Sleep Foundation, our bodies have internal thermostats, and when we go to bed, our brain sets this temperature to a few degrees lower than usual. A slight drop in core temp will make you fall asleep faster, but if it's too hot or too cold, your body may struggle, causing disrupted sleep.

It is recommended to keep your bedroom temperature between 66 degrees and 70 degrees Fahrenheit. You may need to experiment with different temperatures, clothing, and bedding to know what is ideal for you.

Create Darkness

Even a little bit of light can disrupt your sleep, so it's important to make your bedroom as dark as possible. This means blocking out any light sources, including streetlights, electronic devices, and even the moon. Use blackout curtains or shades to keep your bedroom dark, and consider using a sleep mask if necessary. Your brain will naturally produce more melatonin when it's dark, which can help you fall asleep faster and stay asleep longer.

Comfy Bedding

Investing in a quality mattress, pillow, and blanket can make a world of difference in your sleep quality. Old and worn-out pillows and mattresses can affect your sleep and cause back and neck issues. A comfortable and supportive mattress can provide a better sleep surface and reduce pressure points. A good pillow can help keep your neck and spine aligned, and a cozy blanket can make you feel more relaxed and secure.

Relaxing Colors

The colors in your bedroom can also affect your mood and sleep quality. Opt for soothing and relaxing colors, such as blues, greens, and soft neutrals, which can create a calming and serene environment. Avoid bright or bold colors, as they can be too stimulating and prevent you from relaxing. Consider adding accent pillows, rugs, or curtains in calming colors to create a peaceful atmosphere.

Remember, your bedroom should be a place of rest, not stress. So, take the time to make your bedroom a sleep-friendly space and enjoy the benefits of a good night's sleep. Use the Sleep Sanctuary Checklist on the following page to assess your sleep space and plan out a relaxing Sleep Sanctuary.

Action Item: Sleep Sanctuary Checklist

Following, you will find your Sleep Sanctuary Checklist to help you design your perfect sleep environment. While some suggestions like investing in new bedding or repainting might take time, this week, zero in on adjusting room temperature, ensuring darkness, decluttering, and reserving your bedroom solely for sleep. Prioritizing these straightforward changes can profoundly enhance your sleep environment. Refer back to this checklist each night before you wind down for bed.

Sleep Sanctuary Checklist

How can you create a space of calm and tranquility?

My bedroom is clutter free: Yes / No

My bedroom is completely dark at bedtime: Yes / No

My bedroom is cool and comfortable (60-68 F):   Yes / No

I refrain from watching TV, scrolling, checking emails, working, and similar activities while in bed: Yes / No

My sleep partners (significant other, child, pet) do not disrupt me when I am sleeping: Yes / No

I feel relaxed and ready to sleep when in my room: Yes / No

My bedding (mattress, pillows, blankets) are in good shape and comfortable for me: Yes / No

My plan for turning any "No" into a "Yes"

DAY 6

Routines and Rituals

Imagine finishing a whirlwind day, and as soon as your head hits the pillow, you're instantly whisked away into deep, restorative sleep. Sounds dreamy, right? Having a consistent bedtime routine is a great way to help you wind down, relax, and prepare your body for sleep. Personally, I look forward to my nightly ritual and will even try to adhere to it when I am on vacation.

Today we will learn a few ideas you might want to try. But first, fill out your sleep journal on the next page!

Morning Sleep Journal

Complete this each morning to see the impact on your daily sleep!

Today's Date: _____   Bedtime Last Night: _____

How well did you fall asleep?

___ Easily   ___ It took a while   ___ It was difficult

Describe what it was like falling asleep:

Did you wake up and struggle to fall back asleep?

___ Not at all   ___ Once or twice   ___ Multiple times

Describe your experience:

Wake-Up Time: _____   Total Hours of Sleep _____

How did you feel after waking up?

___ Refreshed   ___ Just okay   ___ Tired

Notes:

Get a Head Start On Tomorrow

Having to rush around with morning chores like picking out your clothes, preparing lunches, and packing up your day's necessities will only cause you more stress. Why not take them on as part of your evening routine? It might sound counter-intuitive, but you'll be thanking yourself in the morning when you have a head start on your day. Remember, a great night's sleep begins when you wake up. Don't start your day off in a tizzy.

Jot It Down

Now, let's discuss the power of making a to-do list for the following day. It's like a brain dump that helps clear your mind before bedtime. By jotting down all the tasks you need to tackle the next day, you free up mental space and reduce the stress of trying to remember everything.

Reflecting On Your Day

Journaling can be another calming way to wind down. You could write about your day, express gratitude for the good moments you experienced, or simply write about anything that comes to mind. Journaling can be an excellent way to process thoughts and feelings, allowing your mind to relax.

Settle Down with a Nice Book

A bit of leisurely reading or engaging in a relaxing hobby can also signal to your brain that it's time to unwind. Just make sure the lights are dim to help trigger melatonin production. Also, avoid any books that may be overly stimulating or have disturbing subjects. A dreamy romance novel may do the trick.

Soak the Day Away

How about a warm, soothing bath with Epsom salts? It will help you unwind, and the magnesium in Epsom salts can also help promote a good night's sleep. Plus, it's the perfect time to integrate your skincare routine. I also like adding lavender essential oil to my bath for relaxation. A little self-care can go a long way in signaling to your brain that it's time to rest.

Calm Your Mind

If you find your mind racing with thoughts from the day or are already planning for the next, please introduce a short meditation session into your winding-down routine. Just a few minutes of meditation can make a world of difference. It's all about focusing your mind and letting go of the day's stress. We will dive into some apps for this in a future section. Whether you're a seasoned meditator or a curious newbie, taking this time to be present simply can transition your mind and body into a restful state.

Remember, these are suggestions, and everyone is different! Experiment with these ideas and find out what works best for you. The goal here is to create a routine that you look forward to that signals to your body and mind, "It's time to wind down, relax, and sleep." Enjoy the process of crafting your personal bedtime ritual, and your sleep will thank you!

Are you ready to put this information into practice? Get ready for your next action item, designing your personal wind-down routine.

Action Item: Design Your Perfect Routine

Use the Wind-Down template on the next page to design your personal wind-down routine.

No need to rush.

Ease into it by establishing a schedule. Then, experiment with relaxing activities throughout the program.

My Wind-Down Routine

Create a list of activities as well as a start time. Here are a few prompts to get you started discovering what will work best for you.

I will begin my wind-down routine at...

I will turn off my electronics at...

I will dim the lights at...

Some relaxing activities I can do are...

Describe your wind-down routine:

DAY 7

Check-In: How Did You Do?

Congratulations! You've just completed the first week of your sleep transformation journey. It's now time to pause, reflect, and assess how you've done so far.

Did you take your baseline sleep assessment? This initial step is crucial in understanding where you're starting from. It's like your 'before' snapshot that you can look back on and compare as we progress.

Have you taken the sleep oath seriously? Remember, this is your pledge to prioritize sleep as a non-negotiable element of your health and well-being.

Are you sticking with your sleep schedule? The predictability of going to bed and waking up at the same time each day can significantly impact your sleep quality.

How's your sleep sanctuary coming along? The environment where you sleep can either promote or hinder restful sleep. Have you noticed any improvements?

Do you have a wind-down routine? What relaxing activities have you incorporated?

39

Lastly, have you kept tracking your sleep in the morning journal? This tool is an integral part of the program, helping you to understand your sleep patterns and make connections with your daily activities.

Take a few minutes now to reflect on these questions, jotting down any observations or insights in your journal. Remember, this isn't about perfection but progress. Any steps, no matter how small, towards improving your sleep are victories to celebrate!

With the first week behind us, we're ready to embark on the next stage of your journey-connecting the dots. Get ready to become a sleep detective! Let's keep this momentum going and continue to work towards conquering your insomnia!

Morning Sleep Journal

Complete this each morning to see the impact on your daily sleep!

Today's Date: _____   Bedtime Last Night: _____

How well did you fall asleep?

___ Easily   ____ It took a while   ____ It was difficult

Describe what it was like falling asleep:

Did you wake up and struggle to fall back asleep?

___ Not at all   ____ Once or twice   ____ Multiple times

Describe your experience:

Wake-Up Time: _____   Total Hours of Sleep _____

How did you feel after waking up?

___ Refreshed   ____ Just okay   ____ Tired

Notes:

WEEK 2

Becoming a Sleep Detective

Congratulations on wrapping up the first week of your sleep journey! You're making incredible strides towards reclaiming your sleep! We'll build on this strong foundation as we gear up for week 2. Each day, we'll explore the various activities and habits affecting your sleep quality.

We will also introduce the Evening Journal to enhance your sleep tracking. By week's end, you'll have mapped out your sleep landscape, setting the stage for you to decode your sleep patterns effectively. Get ready to become a Sleep Detective!

DAY 8

Perfect Sleep Starts the Moment You Awake

Cracking the code for impeccable sleep isn't just about the moments before you tuck yourself in. Believe it or not, the secret to blissful slumber begins the moment your eyes flutter open with the first light of day. It's a symphony of decisions we make, consciously or otherwise, from the minute we stir to the second we surrender to the night. This week you will learn how tweaking these everyday habits, even subtly, can dramatically transform your sleepscape. Let's begin by exploring how something as basic as light can profoundly influence your sleep.

Before we begin, remember to complete your morning sleep journal on the next page.

Morning Sleep Journal

Complete this each morning to see the impact on your daily sleep!

Today's Date: _____   Bedtime Last Night: _____

How well did you fall asleep?

___ Easily   ___ It took a while   ___ It was difficult

Describe what it was like falling asleep:

Did you wake up and struggle to fall back asleep?

___ Not at all   ___ Once or twice   ___ Multiple times

Describe your experience:

Wake-Up Time: _____   Total Hours of Sleep _____

How did you feel after waking up?

___ Refreshed   ___ Just okay   ___ Tired

Notes:

What Would Laura Ingalls Do?

Before the widespread availability of electricity, people primarily relied on natural light to rule their day. Let's take one of my favorite shows, "Little House on the Prairie," which was set in the late 1800s. The Ingalls family's lives revolved around the natural patterns of daylight and darkness. They woke up with the sunrise and spent a good part of their day outside in the natural light, keeping them alert and energized.

As the sun began to set, they relaxed and spent quality time together under the warm glow of lanterns, candles, and fireplaces. These natural sources of light emitted a warm, dim glow that had minimal impact on their natural sleep patterns.

As the evening progressed, their natural production of melatonin increased, preparing their bodies for rest. They went to bed shortly after sunset, enjoying a full night of restorative sleep. They woke up refreshed and ready to begin another day.

Fast-forward to today.

With the advent of electricity and the widespread use of artificial lighting, our exposure to light and darkness has changed dramatically. Mostly, we spend our days inside under the harsh illumination of blue light. The blue light emitted by our electronic devices has been shown to have a particularly strong impact on our sleep-wake cycle. Exposure to blue light in the evening can interfere with our natural sleep patterns, making it more difficult to fall asleep and stay asleep throughout the night.

Adjusting the timing and quality of your light exposure is imperative to setting your circadian clock and getting your sleep on track.

Tips to Get Started

It is important to think about both the daytime and evening impact of light on your sleep. Light can be an asset or a weakness in creating a healthy sleep routine.

Daytime

Prioritize natural daylight: Try to step outside within the first hour of awakening. Enjoy your morning coffee outside, take a walk (one of the many benefits of having a dog), or bask in the daylight for 10 to 20 minutes. Longer on cloudy days.

Invest in a Light Box: Sometimes getting early morning sun is easier said than done (I know this firsthand). Living in Michigan (especially in the winter) and waking up several hours before sunrise makes getting my morning light challenging. To help combat this, I use a light box that mimics natural sunlight. I sit in front of my light box while drinking my morning coffee or getting ready for work.

Consider using a sunrise alarm clock: These devices simulate a natural sunrise, gradually increasing the light in your room to help you wake up more gently and in tune with your circadian rhythm. Some models even incorporate soundscapes, such as the lovely sound of chirping birds.

Spend time outdoors during the day: Spending time outdoors (even in the winter) will help relieve stress and set you up for a great night's sleep. If you are stuck in an office all day, try to take your breaks outside or sit near a window.

Evening

Managing your evening light exposure is equally important for your sleep. Your brain will naturally produce more melatonin when it's dark, which can help you fall asleep faster and stay asleep longer.

Dim the lights

Ideally, begin to turn down the lights a couple of hours before bedtime. Candles and a fireplace are nice alternatives (just be sure to snuff them out before you go to sleep). If not, you can also consider investing in orange or red-colored light bulbs as an alternative to blue-emitting light.

Limit screen time before bed

Binging on your favorite television series before bed? Scrolling through Instagram to unwind? I get it. The evening may be the only time to have for yourself. Unfortunately, these nightly rituals may be causing havoc on your sleep. Studies show that exposure to the blue light expressed by electronic devices in the evening hours results in a 25% reduction in melatonin production. Try shutting off your devices 1–2 hours before bedtime. Alternatively, try blue-light-blocking glasses when you must use screens. Stay away from disturbing or triggering media that will trigger your stress response!

Action Item: Evening Sleep Journal

It's time to put on your detective hat! Now that you are beginning to understand your current sleep patterns, it's time to connect the dots. Your Evening Sleep Journal will help you do just that. By adjusting the timing of your daily routines and understanding their impact, you'll optimize your sleep.

Every evening, note your activities, meals, and moods, and then analyze this data against your sleep patterns. Over time, you might start seeing patterns. Perhaps you'll discover that you struggle to fall asleep after a late-night meal or find it hard to stay asleep after your evening glass of wine. We will discuss how these activities may impact your sleep throughout the week.

Use your journal to jot down any patterns or connections you notice between your daily routines and your sleep quality. With this critical insight, you'll be well on your way to figuring out how to enhance your sleep. Would you be able to change the timing of your routines? Embrace new habits? Remember, understanding your sleep is the first step to improving it. Let's connect those dots and set you on a path to better sleep.

Evening Sleep Journal

Incorporate this journal into your evening wind-down routine.

Today's Date: _____

Write down the time/description for each item.

Caffeine	
Supplements	
Medications	
Exercise	
Evening Meal	
Snacks	
Beverages	
Alcohol	
Naps	

My Sleepiness Level Today (Low / Medium / High)

My Stress Level Today (Low / Medium / High)

Can you make any connections to activities that impacted sleep?

DAY 9

Do You Caffeinate?

"Oh, what a beautiful morning; oh, what a beautiful day; until I've had my coffee, you'd better stay out of my way". I saw this saying on a coffee mug and laughed. "Yep, that's me". The first thing I do every morning is turn on the coffee pot I routinely set up the night before. And although I do not plan on giving coffee up anytime soon, I do know that if I am not careful it can wreak havoc on my sleep.

We will learn the reasons why, but first, remember to complete your morning sleep journal on the next page.

Morning Sleep Journal

Complete this each morning to see the impact on your daily sleep!

Today's Date: _____   Bedtime Last Night: _____

How well did you fall asleep?

___ Easily   ____ It took a while   ____ It was difficult

Describe what it was like falling asleep:

Did you wake up and struggle to fall back asleep?

___ Not at all   ____ Once or twice   ____ Multiple times

Describe your experience:

Wake-Up Time: _____   Total Hours of Sleep _____

How did you feel after waking up?

___ Refreshed   ____ Just okay   ____ Tired

Notes:

The Impact of Caffeine

Caffeine is a stimulant and can trigger your stress hormones (cortisol and adrenaline). Cortisol will suppress your melatonin (you will hear me say this often). Too much caffeine can increase anxiety, which will also ruin your sleep.

Caffeine also blocks your adenosine receptors. Remember, adenosine is the chemical in your brain that gradually induces sleep pressure throughout the day. By blocking the receptors, you will decrease your feeling of sleepiness when it comes time to tuck in. But never fear. I am not suggesting you give up your morning brew. Just be mindful of when and how much you consume. Caffeine has a half-life of 6 to 8 hours. This means that if you have a cup of coffee at 3:00, half of the caffeine is still in your system at 11:00 at night.

And the rate at which people metabolize caffeine varies from person to person. I have friends who can easily fall asleep after having an espresso while watching TV at night. Others who imbibe in even the slightest bit of caffeine during the day will no doubt be tossing and turning throughout the night.

Tolerance Levels and Quantity

Your tolerance can also change as you age. I know this has been the case for me. Topping off my dinner with a cup of coffee was never an issue in my 20s. As the years passed, my cutoff times became earlier and earlier. I went from any time to 4:00 to 1:00, to 11:00. Now, if I have coffee past 10:00 in the morning, I will certainly be staring at my ceiling fan when my head hits the pillow.

Coffee is not the only place where caffeine can hide. You will also find it in various beverages, foods, supplements, and medications.

- **Coffee** - An 8-ounce cup has approximately 95 mg
- **Espresso** - 1 shot or 1.5 ounces, contains about 65 mg
- **Decaffeinated coffee** - Contains about 4 mg of caffeine
- **Tea** - 1 cup of black tea contains about 47 mg and, green tea contains about 28 mg. Decaffeinated tea contains 2 mg. Pro tip: herbal tea contains none!
- **Soda** - A 12-ounce can of cola contains about 40 mg of caffeine. Mountain Dew contains 55 mg!
- **Chocolate (cacao)** - 1 ounce of dark chocolate contains about 24 mg. Milk chocolate contains one-quarter of that amount.
- **Energy drinks** - 8 ounces of an energy drink contains about 85 mg and a 2-ounce shot contains about 200 mg!

If you think caffeine may be robbing you of sleep, you can experiment by giving yourself a caffeine curfew or giving it up altogether.

When you are weaning off of coffee, try gradually decreasing your caffeine consumption by cutting it with decaf. Begin with half of each and increase the decaf amount each day until you are on full decaf. You can also start using alternatives to kick the habit.

Caffeine Alternatives

- **Herbal tea** - besides being caffeine-free, herbal teas have many other stress-relieving and health benefits.
- **Dandy blend** - a great coffee alternative made from dandelion and chicory root extract.
- **Hot lemon water** - beginning and ending your day with hot lemon water has many benefits, including aiding digestion and boosting immunity.
- **Golden milk latte** - made with coconut milk, turmeric, and other spices, this creamy drink is great in the morning or in the evening to help wind down your day.

Whether you limit yourself to a morning jolt, a 3:00 pick-me-up, or numerous "coffee meetings" throughout the day, monitoring your caffeine can be an important component of fixing your sleep. Track it in your Evening Sleep Journal!

Evening Sleep Journal

Incorporate this journal into your evening wind-down routine.

Today's Date: _____

Write down the time/description for each item.

Caffeine	
Supplements	
Medications	
Exercise	
Evening Meal	
Snacks	
Beverages	
Alcohol	
Naps	

My Sleepiness Level Today (Low / Medium / High)

My Stress Level Today (Low / Medium / High)

Can you make any connections to activities that impacted sleep?

DAY 10

Time Your Workouts

We all know that exercise is good for us. I have been working out since Jane Fonda donned her first pair of leg warmers. Over the years, I have experimented with everything from yoga to CrossFit. As I have gotten older, and due to some health issues, I have been more focused on walking, Zumba, strength training, and yoga. But even with these seemingly low-impact forms of exercise, I still must be mindful of timing as it relates to my sleep. There is a reason for this.

Before we get to that, take some time to do your Morning Sleep Journal for today.

Morning Sleep Journal

Complete this each morning to see the impact on your daily sleep!

Today's Date: _____   Bedtime Last Night: _____

How well did you fall asleep?

___ Easily   ____ It took a while   ____ It was difficult

Describe what it was like falling asleep:

Did you wake up and struggle to fall back asleep?

___ Not at all   ____ Once or twice   ____ Multiple times

Describe your experience:

Wake-Up Time: _____   Total Hours of Sleep _____

How did you feel after waking up?

___ Refreshed   ____ Just okay   ____ Tired

Notes:

Why Timing Matters

Research has shown that exercising too close to bedtime can disrupt our circadian rhythm and make it harder to fall asleep. This is because exercise raises our body temperature, which can interfere with the body's natural cooling process that occurs during sleep. Some forms of exercise, such as cardio and strength training, can also increase your cortisol, hence down-regulating your melatonin production.

So, if you are dealing with sleep issues, aim to exercise earlier in the day. Research has shown that exercising in the morning or early afternoon can help regulate our circadian rhythm and promote healthy sleep patterns. Additionally, exercising in the morning can help reduce stress and anxiety, which can also contribute to insomnia. This is not to say that an evening walk or yoga session is off the table. Try to schedule your major sweat session for earlier in the day.

Be sure to track your exercise timing in your Evening Sleep Journal.

Evening Sleep Journal

Incorporate this journal into your evening wind-down routine.

Today's Date: _____

Write down the time/description for each item.

Caffeine	
Supplements	
Medications	
Exercise	
Evening Meal	
Snacks	
Beverages	
Alcohol	
Naps	

My Sleepiness Level Today (Low / Medium / High)

My Stress Level Today (Low / Medium / High)

Can you make any connections to activities that impacted sleep?

DAY 11

Sync Your Supper

Think about the last time you had a hefty meal just before bed. Remember the tossing, turning, and that unsettling feeling in your stomach? If you're nodding your head, we're right on the same page. Through the insights gained from journaling, I've discovered a clear link between late-night dinners and my restless nights.

Speaking of which, take some time to complete your Morning Sleep Journal before we dive deeper into this topic.

Morning Sleep Journal

Complete this each morning to see the impact on your daily sleep!

Today's Date: _____   Bedtime Last Night: _____

How well did you fall asleep?

___ Easily   ____ It took a while   ____ It was difficult

Describe what it was like falling asleep:

Did you wake up and struggle to fall back asleep?

___ Not at all   ____ Once or twice   ____ Multiple times

Describe your experience:

Wake-Up Time: _____   Total Hours of Sleep _____

How did you feel after waking up?

___ Refreshed   ____ Just okay   ____ Tired

Notes:

Digestion and Sleep

Our bodies need to kick up their heels and relax at bedtime, not work overtime on digestion. While meal timing plays a pivotal role, let's not sidestep the quantity and the 'fullness' factor. Gobbling down a mountain-sized dinner can feel like you've dropped an anchor in your stomach. An overfull belly not only makes it uncomfortable to find that perfect sleep position but also burdens your digestive system. When the body should be shifting into rest mode, it's instead grappling with the hefty task of breaking down that banquet you consumed.

It's all about balance – eating enough to feel satisfied without crossing into the territory of feeling like an overstuffed pillow. So, as you reconsider your dinner timing, also keep an eye on portion sizes and listen to your body's cues about satiety.

So, here's the game plan: Eat until you feel satisfied, and aim to have your dinner plate cleared at least 2–3 hours before hitting the hay. This gives your body ample time to process your meal and wind down for the day. It may be a game changer for your sleep quality.

Could your evening feast be the undercover culprit stealing your sleep? Jot down those meal times in your Evening Sleep Journal, and let's play detective.

Evening Sleep Journal

Incorporate this journal into your evening wind-down routine.

Today's Date: _____

Write down the time/description for each item.

Caffeine	
Supplements	
Medications	
Exercise	
Evening Meal	
Snacks	
Beverages	
Alcohol	
Naps	

My Sleepiness Level Today (Low / Medium / High)

My Stress Level Today (Low / Medium / High)

Can you make any connections to activities that impacted sleep?

DAY 12

Pill Timing Tactics

While we take supplements and medications hoping for better health, they can sometimes play unexpected roles in our sleep struggles.

We will review many different supplements and medications that could affect your sleep - and how to manage them for the best possible outcome. Remember what we talked about all the way at the beginning of the book, and consult your doctor about any medication or supplement changes.

First, complete your Morning Sleep Journal on the next page.

Morning Sleep Journal

Complete this each morning to see the impact on your daily sleep!

Today's Date: _____   Bedtime Last Night: _____

How well did you fall asleep?

___ Easily   ____ It took a while   ____ It was difficult

Describe what it was like falling asleep:

Did you wake up and struggle to fall back asleep?

___ Not at all   ____ Once or twice   ____ Multiple times

Describe your experience:

Wake-Up Time: _____   Total Hours of Sleep _____

How did you feel after waking up?

___ Refreshed   ____ Just okay   ____ Tired

Notes:

Supplements

Picture supplements like a seesaw. On one end, there's a crowd of vitamin deficiencies that could be ruining your sleep. On the other end, there are supplements that could be doing the same thing. Here's a bit of a breakdown of supplements with potential sleep-stealing side effects.

Vitamin D

Don't photobomb your sleep! Vitamin D is known as the "sunshine vitamin" because your body typically produces it in response to sunlight. Taking it later in the day could mimic sunlight exposure and interfere with your melatonin production. To be safe, aim to take your daily dose in the morning.

Weight Loss Pills

Think of these as the little energizer bunnies. Many of them are pumped full of caffeine and other stimulants to keep hunger at bay. But when night falls, they're still hopping around, keeping you awake.

Vitamins B5, B6, B12, and B-Complex

Picture these B vitamins as the party guests who just won't leave. They're fantastic for boosting your energy levels during the day, but when it's time for bed, they're still wired and keeping you up.

Multivitamins

These are like a little mystery box. They may have a mix of vitamins that mess with your sleep, and some even include additives that could do the same.

Glucosamine & Chondroitin

These are the good guys, the peacekeepers. They work to relieve joint pain, improve joint function, and reduce inflammation. But strangely enough, they're also listed as potential insomnia culprits. Scientists aren't quite sure why, but it's worth considering.

If you think your supplements are sleep bandits, try taking them in the morning or earlier in the day. Play detective with your supplement routine to see what works best for you.

Medications

Could it be that your prescriptions are moonlighting as secret sleep saboteurs? You might be wrestling with your sheets, watching the clock inch towards dawn, while your medication quietly undermines your good night's rest. According to AARP, several kinds of drugs have a notorious reputation for instigating sleep issues

Alpha-blockers

Examples: Prazosin (Minipress), Terazosin (Hytrin)
Alpha-blockers can decrease REM sleep and increase daytime sleepiness, leading to nighttime sleeplessness.

Beta-blockers

Examples: Atenolol (Tenormin), Metoprolol (Lopressor, Toprol-XL)
These medications have been linked to sleep disturbances and nightmares, as they can reduce melatonin production.

Corticosteroids

Examples: Prednisone, Cortisone
Corticosteroids can mimic the adrenal glands' effects, impacting stress and relaxation regulation, affecting sleep.

SSRI Antidepressants

Examples: Fluoxetine (Prozac), Sertraline (Zoloft)
While the exact mechanism is unclear, SSRIs have been associated with agitation, sleeplessness, and mild tremors in some individuals.

ACE Inhibitors

Examples: Lisinopril (Prinivil, Zestril), Ramipril (Altace)
Frequent coughing and increased potassium production, which may lead to diarrhea, cramps, and joint, bone, and muscle pain, can keep you awake at night.

ARBs (Angiotensin II Receptor Blockers)

Examples: Losartan (Cozaar), Valsartan (Diovan)
Like ACE inhibitors, ARBs can cause a buildup of potassium, triggering pain and making it hard to sleep.

H1 Antagonists

Examples: Diphenhydramine (Benadryl), Loratadine (Claritin)
H1 antagonists block acetylcholine, a neurotransmitter that can cause anxiety and insomnia when disrupted.

Statins

Examples: Atorvastatin (Lipitor), Simvastatin (Zocor)
Muscle pain, a common side effect of statins, can make sleeping difficult. Fat-soluble statins are more likely to cause insomnia and nightmares as they penetrate cell membranes and cross the blood-brain barrier.

Next Steps

If you suspect your medications or supplements might be affecting your sleep, consult with your healthcare provider. They may recommend a replacement or a change in the time you take your medication. Remember, never discontinue any medication without discussing it with your doctor first.

Start tracking your supplement and medication timing in your Evening Sleep Journal.

Evening Sleep Journal

Incorporate this journal into your evening wind-down routine.

Today's Date: _____

Write down the time/description for each item.

Caffeine	
Supplements	
Medications	
Exercise	
Evening Meal	
Snacks	
Beverages	
Alcohol	
Naps	

My Sleepiness Level Today (Low / Medium / High)

My Stress Level Today (Low / Medium / High)

Can you make any connections to activities that impacted sleep?

DAY 13

Wine-ing Down?

Ah, my nightly ritual... a nice glass of wine to help me relax and shake off the day. I really looked forward to it. And it did help me to fall asleep for a bit. Unfortunately, I would wake up in the middle of the night, unable to fall back asleep.

There are some important reasons why this is happening in your body, but first, fill out your Morning Sleep Journal.

Morning Sleep Journal

Complete this each morning to see the impact on your daily sleep!

Today's Date: _____   Bedtime Last Night: _____

How well did you fall asleep?

___ Easily   ____ It took a while   ____ It was difficult

Describe what it was like falling asleep:

Did you wake up and struggle to fall back asleep?

___ Not at all   ____ Once or twice   ____ Multiple times

Describe your experience:

Wake-Up Time: _____   Total Hours of Sleep _____

How did you feel after waking up?

___ Refreshed   ____ Just okay   ____ Tired

Notes:

Alcohol and Sleep

Alcohol is a sedative and will certainly help you to feel drowsy. However, once your liver metabolizes alcohol, there will be a rebound effect of alertness, disrupting sleep cycles during the second half of the night. Even if you do sleep through the night, you may feel tired and spacey the next day.

There are other reasons why alcohol may disrupt your sleep. Alcohol is a diuretic, which means you may dehydrate during the night (not to mention having to get up to pee numerous times). It also relaxes your throat muscles, which can contribute to snoring and sleep apnea.

If you think alcohol may be playing a role in your sleep issues, you do have options. You can give it up completely and maybe try a nice cup of chamomile tea or a golden milk latte. Or you simply give yourself an alcohol curfew. Ideally, stop alcohol consumption at least 3 hours before bed. For some people, it may be longer. I know that if I drink past 4:00, I will have disrupted sleep. Experiment and track in your Sleep Journal to see what works best for you.

Last, but definitely not least, if you are experiencing alcohol dependency, please consult with your doctor.

Evening Sleep Journal

Incorporate this journal into your evening wind-down routine.

Today's Date: _____

Write down the time/description for each item.

Caffeine	
Supplements	
Medications	
Exercise	
Evening Meal	
Snacks	
Beverages	
Alcohol	
Naps	

My Sleepiness Level Today (Low / Medium / High)

My Stress Level Today (Low / Medium / High)

Can you make any connections to activities that impacted sleep?

75

DAY 14
Week 2 Check-In

Congratulations on successfully navigating through week 2! You've taken some significant strides in your journey towards mastering sleep. Dialing in your daily routine and beginning to connect the dots with sleep bandits are substantial steps toward uncovering the secrets of your sleep patterns.

But before we do, take a moment to reflect on the changes you've implemented so far:

- How is your wind-down routine working for you?
- Have you been able to stick to a consistent sleep schedule?
- Are you beginning to associate the timing of your daily activities with your sleep quality?

Remember, this journey is about discovery and adaptation. Keep up the excellent work, and gear up for week 3, where we dive into the realms of our minds and emotions. Here, we often find the root causes of our sleep disturbances - stress, negative thought patterns, and an overactive mind! Get ready to learn various stress management and relaxation techniques that will help you clear the way to peace and tranquility. And be sure to complete your Morning and Evening Sleep Journal today!

Morning Sleep Journal

Complete this each morning to see the impact on your daily sleep!

Today's Date: _____   Bedtime Last Night: _____

How well did you fall asleep?

___ Easily   ____ It took a while   ____ It was difficult

Describe what it was like falling asleep:

Did you wake up and struggle to fall back asleep?

___ Not at all   ____ Once or twice   ____ Multiple times

Describe your experience:

Wake-Up Time: _____   Total Hours of Sleep _____

How did you feel after waking up?

___ Refreshed   ____ Just okay   ____ Tired

Notes:

Evening Sleep Journal

Incorporate this journal into your evening wind-down routine.

Today's Date: _____

Write down the time/description for each item.

Caffeine	
Supplements	
Medications	
Exercise	
Evening Meal	
Snacks	
Beverages	
Alcohol	
Naps	

My Sleepiness Level Today (Low / Medium / High)

My Stress Level Today (Low / Medium / High)

Can you make any connections to activities that impacted sleep?

WEEK 3

Master Mind Management

Whether it is ruminating over sending that snarky email, worrying about my aging parents, or stressing over my never-ending to-do list, racing thoughts have disrupted many a night's sleep for me. Why is it that my worry machine goes into full gear once my head hits the pillow?

We tend to worry more at bedtime because our minds are more relaxed and less occupied with the distractions of daily activities. This can make it easier for thoughts and worries to surface and become magnified in our minds, leading to anxiety and stress.

This week, we will explore these and other internal sources of missing sleep. Better yet, we will discover strategies to manage these stressors.

DAY 15

Stress, Worry, and Racing Thoughts!

Bedtime, for some, has become associated with worry and anxiety. If you frequently find yourself worrying at night, your brain may begin to connect the process of getting ready for bed with these anxious thoughts, leading to a cycle of worry and disrupted sleep.

Moreover, being in a dark and quiet environment can increase our sense of vulnerability and make it harder to calm down and fall asleep. So, it's no surprise that many people struggle with falling asleep or staying asleep due to worrying or anxiety.

Stress, in general, will have a big impact on your ability to get a good night's sleep. When we experience stress, our bodies release cortisol, which activates our fight-or-flight response. This is a survival instinct that's meant to help us become more alert to potential threats. But the problem is that our bodies can't always distinguish between a real threat and something that we're just imagining. Even if we're worried, our bodies still react as though there's a real danger. This can lead to racing thoughts and anxiety, making it even more difficult to relax. It's important to find ways to manage stress in order to get a good night's sleep.

Morning Sleep Journal

Complete this each morning to see the impact on your daily sleep!

Today's Date: _____   Bedtime Last Night: _____

How well did you fall asleep?

___ Easily   ____ It took a while   ____ It was difficult

Describe what it was like falling asleep:

Did you wake up and struggle to fall back asleep?

___ Not at all   ____ Once or twice   ____ Multiple times

Describe your experience:

Wake-Up Time: _____   Total Hours of Sleep _____

How did you feel after waking up?

___ Refreshed   ____ Just okay   ____ Tired

Notes:

Forms of Stress

Stress can come in many forms, and it affects the body in different ways. Understanding where your stress comes from and how it impacts you personally can help you minimize the effect on your sleep.

Which of these forms of stress resonate the most for you?

Acute Stress

Acute stress is a short-term response to a specific triggering event, such as the jitters before a big presentation or the sudden shock from a minor car accident. It's the body's immediate reaction, sparking the 'fight or flight' response. While it can induce heightened alertness and focus, it can also cause distress, especially if the incidents are frequent.

Then there's episodic acute stress – think of it as acute stress on repeat. This occurs when an individual confronts multiple stress-inducing events quickly, like having a series of job interviews in a week or facing back-to-back deadlines. The repeated nature of this stress type can lead to feelings of constant tension and agitation, making it crucial to manage effectively.

Chronic Stress

Chronic stress is a relentless strain that persists over extended periods, often stemming from enduring challenges in life. Whether it's a high-pressure job, ongoing family issues, or a challenging relationship, chronic stress can have long-term health implications if not addressed, including sleep disruptions, weakened immune function, and increased risk for certain diseases.

Physiological Stress

This type of stress arises from physical traumas or ailments that the body endures. Examples include recovering from surgery, battling a chronic illness, or pushing through a rigorous physical challenge. The body's reaction to these stressors can be varied, from increased heart rate to the release of specific hormones that affect mood and energy levels.

Psychological Stress

Rooted in the mind, psychological stress can be triggered by a myriad of emotional or mental challenges. Anxiety, depression, grief, or even intense bouts of anger can incite this form of stress. It's not just about the triggering events, but also about how an individual perceives and processes these emotional experiences, which can further intensify the stress response.

Traumatic Stress

This type of stress emerges in the aftermath of encountering deeply distressing events, such as natural calamities, acts of violence, or intense combat situations. The magnitude of these events often leaves an individual grappling with intense emotional, physical, and mental reactions. Memories of the trauma can resurface unpredictably, often triggering flashbacks or nightmares. The profound nature of traumatic stress might necessitate therapeutic interventions or counseling to help individuals cope, process, and eventually heal from the harrowing experiences they've endured.

Rumination

Rumination is when someone repetitively and persistently thinks or dwells on the same thoughts, emotions, experiences, or memories, often leading to a negative spiral of emotions and thoughts. It can be caused by stress, anxiety, depression, and negative life events, and even certain personality traits and cognitive factors can contribute to rumination.

Catastrophizing

This cognitive distortion prompts people to jump to the worst possible conclusion after a minor setback. It's like a mental magnifying glass for all things negative, casting shadows much larger than the actual issue. If you've ever had a small disagreement with a friend and then convinced yourself that the friendship is over, you've experienced catastrophizing.

General Anxiety

General anxiety is a persistent feeling of worry, fear, or nervousness. Unlike specific anxieties that relate to situations, general anxiety is chronic, unrelenting, and can be triggered by almost anything. It's like having an alarm system in your brain that's a little too sensitive, ringing the bells and blowing the whistles even when there's no actual danger.

Dealing with Stress and Anxiety

Dealing with stress, anxiety, and negative thought patterns can be challenging, but strategies and techniques such as Reframing, Journaling, Breathwork, and Meditation can help. As you progress through this program, you'll learn how to apply these strategies not just to your sleep but to all areas of your life. After all, better sleep is just one part of the bigger picture: a happier, healthier you.

Beginning tonight, tune into your mind and body when you feel the onset of stress or anxiety. Are you dealing with an acute or chronic stress issue? Are you ruminating or catastrophizing? Can you pinpoint the triggers of your stress? Understanding where your stress is coming from can be helpful when developing coping strategies. Over the next week, you will learn techniques to help calm your mind and relax your body.

To get started, complete your Evening Sleep Journal.

Evening Sleep Journal

Incorporate this journal into your evening wind-down routine.

Today's Date: _____

Write down the time/description for each item.

Caffeine	
Supplements	
Medications	
Exercise	
Evening Meal	
Snacks	
Beverages	
Alcohol	
Naps	

My Sleepiness Level Today (Low / Medium / High)

My Stress Level Today (Low / Medium / High)

Can you make any connections to activities that impacted sleep?

DAY 16

Reframing Techniques for Better Sleep

Does your worry machine go into full gear just as your head hits the pillow? These negative thoughts can exacerbate your sleep problems by increasing stress and anxiety. Cognitive reframing is a powerful technique that can help you recognize and shift these thoughts, leading to a more relaxed state and improved sleep quality.

Following is a step-by-step technique that you can try the next time you begin to experience a negative thought pattern. But first, fill out your Morning Sleep Journal.

Morning Sleep Journal

Complete this each morning to see the impact on your daily sleep!

Today's Date: _____   Bedtime Last Night: _____

How well did you fall asleep?

___ Easily   ____ It took a while   ____ It was difficult

Describe what it was like falling asleep:

Did you wake up and struggle to fall back asleep?

___ Not at all   ____ Once or twice   ____ Multiple times

Describe your experience:

Wake-Up Time: _____   Total Hours of Sleep _____

How did you feel after waking up?

___ Refreshed   ____ Just okay   ____ Tired

Notes:

Reframing Step-By-Step

Step One: Identify Negative Thoughts

- Recognize the thought patterns that are causing stress or anxiety, such as excessive worry or self-criticism.
- Be mindful of the situations or triggers often leading to these negative thoughts.

Step Two: Challenge the Thoughts

- Ask yourself if the negative thought is based on facts or assumptions.
- Consider whether the thought is helpful or harmful to your well-being.
- Look for evidence that contradicts the negative thought.

Step Three: Consider Alternative Perspectives

- Look at different ways to interpret the situation or event that triggered the negative thought.
- Ask yourself how someone else might view the situation, or what advice you would give to a friend in a similar situation.

Step Four: Replace Negative Thoughts with Balanced Thoughts

- Develop a more balanced, realistic perspective by considering alternative viewpoints.
- Replace the negative thought with a more positive or neutral thought that reflects this new perspective.

Putting It Into Practice

Let's look at a personal example.

Step One: Identify the Negative Thought

My son has not responded to my texts all day. Something terrible must have happened (Catastrophizing).

Step Two: Challenge the Thought

Is this the only possible reason that my son may not be responding? Are there alternative explanations?

Step Three: Alternate Perspective

He is probably just busy or out of cell phone range.

Step Four: Reframe

He is most likely fine. It is not like this has not happened before. If something is wrong, I will deal with it in a constructive way.

Action Item: Practice Reframing

Acknowledge your thoughts and emotions without judgment and allow them to pass without engaging in negative self-talk. Treat yourself with kindness and understanding, recognizing that negative thoughts are a normal part of the human experience.

Incorporating reframing techniques into your bedtime routine can help you manage negative thoughts and create a more relaxed mental state, promoting better sleep. It may take time and practice to reframe thoughts effectively, but with consistency, you can develop a more balanced mindset and improve your overall well-being.

Now you can practice this technique. On the next page is a Reframing Worksheet you can use to walk you through each of the four steps. You will also find additional Reframing worksheets in the Resources section of this book, so you can use this strategy whenever you need to.

After completing the reframing practice, be sure to complete your Evening Sleep Journal!

Reframing Worksheet

Use this tool whenever you need help managing stressful thoughts.

Today's Date: _____

Step One: Identify the Negative Thought

What is the negative or recurring thought? What event triggered this thought?

Step Two: Challenge the Thought

Is there any evidence that this is true? Is there evidence that this thought may be false?

Step Three: Reframe the Thought

What is the worst thing that could happen if this thought came true? What is the most likely thing to happen? Is there anything I can do about this? Is there another way to look at this?

Step Four: New Thought

Evening Sleep Journal

Incorporate this journal into your evening wind-down routine.

Today's Date: _____

Write down the time/description for each item.

Caffeine	
Supplements	
Medications	
Exercise	
Evening Meal	
Snacks	
Beverages	
Alcohol	
Naps	

My Sleepiness Level Today (Low / Medium / High)

My Stress Level Today (Low / Medium / High)

Can you make any connections to activities that impacted sleep?

DAY 17

Get It Out of Your Head

Another way to improve sleep quality is by finding ways to clear your mind and manage intrusive thoughts. Today we will explore several techniques, including to-do lists, worry lists, and designated worry time. These strategies for clearing your mind can have an immediate impact on your sleep quality and quantity.

Right now, complete your Morning Sleep Journal, and then we can get to the strategies.

Morning Sleep Journal

Complete this each morning to see the impact on your daily sleep!

Today's Date: _____   Bedtime Last Night: _____

How well did you fall asleep?

___ Easily   ____ It took a while   ____ It was difficult

Describe what it was like falling asleep:

Did you wake up and struggle to fall back asleep?

___ Not at all   ____ Once or twice   ____ Multiple times

Describe your experience:

Wake-Up Time: _____   Total Hours of Sleep _____

How did you feel after waking up?

___ Refreshed   ____ Just okay   ____ Tired

Notes:

To-Do Lists

As previously mentioned, creating a to-do list can help you declutter your mind and organize your thoughts. By writing down your tasks and responsibilities, you can free up mental space, allowing you to relax and focus on sleep. Try these tips for effective to-do lists:

- Write your to-do list before bedtime, so you're not thinking about tasks while trying to sleep.
- Keep your list simple and focused, prioritizing the most important tasks.
- Review your list in the morning to help you start your day with a clear plan.

It is common to get anxious when we think about our endless to-do lists. Writing it down can help. Leave your list within reach in case you wake up in the night and feel the need to add to it.

Be sure to spend time the next day creating a plan to manage your tasks, so you can stop stressing.

Worry Lists

Similar to a to-do list, a worry list is a place to write down your concerns and anxieties. This can help you gain perspective on your worries and prevent them from overwhelming you at bedtime.

Follow these steps to create a worry list:

- Set aside a few minutes each evening to write down your concerns and anxieties.
- Acknowledge each worry and remind yourself that you'll address it at a more appropriate time. (designated worry time).
- Review your worry list during the next day to see if any issues require action or resolution.
- Acknowledge each worry and remind yourself that you'll address it at a more appropriate time (designated worry time).

Designated Worry Time

Designated worry time is a technique that involves setting aside a specific time each day to process your concerns and anxieties. By allocating a designated time to worry, you can train your mind to postpone anxious thoughts until that time, helping you relax and sleep better.

How to Worry On Schedule

Choose a Consistent Time:

Pick a time each day, preferably earlier in the afternoon, to avoid interfering with bedtime. For instance, 3:00 PM when taking a break from work or chores. Mark it on your calendar or set a daily reminder on your phone.

Find a Quiet Place:

Locate a quiet space where you won't be disturbed. This could be a corner in your living room, a park bench, or even your car.

Set a Timer:

Allow yourself 15–30 minutes. You can adjust this time based on your needs but try not to extend it too long. The goal is to have a focused session without it consuming a large part of your day.

Journal Your Thoughts:

You may find it helpful to write down your worries. For instance, you might write:

- "I'm concerned about my presentation tomorrow."
- "I'm feeling overwhelmed with my to-do list."
- "I'm worried about my child's performance in school."

Once you've listed your worries, brainstorm potential solutions or next steps, even if they're small.

Visualization:

Imagine placing your worries into a box or floating them down a river. This visualization can help in compartmentalizing and letting go.

Conclude Your Session:

Once the timer rings, take a few deep breaths and commit to leaving your worries behind until the next designated time. Remind yourself that you've given these concerns their due attention for today.

Post-Worry Activities:

When your designated worry time is over, engage in an activity that you enjoy or find relaxing. This could be reading a book, taking a walk, or listening to music. This transition helps shift your mindset and offers a break from the intensity of your session.

Over time, you may find that your worries become less consuming, or you might discover practical solutions to the concerns that once seemed insurmountable. Remember, like any skill, mastering designated worry time takes practice.

Take a few minutes to complete your Evening Sleep Journal now, and tomorrow we will talk about making journaling even more effective.

Evening Sleep Journal

Incorporate this journal into your evening wind-down routine.

Today's Date: _____

Write down the time/description for each item.

Caffeine	
Supplements	
Medications	
Exercise	
Evening Meal	
Snacks	
Beverages	
Alcohol	
Naps	

My Sleepiness Level Today (Low / Medium / High)

My Stress Level Today (Low / Medium / High)

Can you make any connections to activities that impacted sleep?

DAY 18

The Transformative Power of Journaling

Journaling is much more than putting pen to paper; it's a therapeutic journey of self-reflection and discovery. If done consistently, this powerful exercise can become your secret weapon against sleepless nights filled with relentless rumination.

The act of journaling goes beyond merely jotting down events. It allows you to dissect, process, and, most importantly, release the day's accumulated mental clutter. And the beauty of it? The more you dive into this practice, the more you uncover about yourself — patterns of thought, triggers of stress, and nuggets of self-awareness.

Start with your Morning Sleep Journal, and then I will share some of my most powerful journaling tips.

Morning Sleep Journal

Complete this each morning to see the impact on your daily sleep!

Today's Date: _____   Bedtime Last Night: _____

How well did you fall asleep?

___ Easily   ____ It took a while   ____ It was difficult

Describe what it was like falling asleep:

Did you wake up and struggle to fall back asleep?

___ Not at all   ____ Once or twice   ____ Multiple times

Describe your experience:

Wake-Up Time: _____   Total Hours of Sleep _____

How did you feel after waking up?

___ Refreshed   ____ Just okay   ____ Tired

Notes:

Embrace the Ritual

Dedicate a quiet space and a specific time for this activity. Making it consistent can enhance its therapeutic effect.

Dig Deeper

Instead of merely cataloging events, delve into how they made you feel, why they affected you so, and how you can handle similar situations better in the future.

Practice Gratitude

Concluding your journaling session by noting three things you're grateful for can shift your focus from anxiety to appreciation, paving the way for a peaceful night's sleep.

Let It Flow

There's no right or wrong way to journal. Whether it's bullet points, doodles, or long-form writing, do what feels right for you. Remember, this space is just for you, free from judgment.

Reflecting on my journey, I discovered something that changed my outlook. Most anxieties that occupied my mind never actually materialized. It's a stark reminder that the stories we weave in our minds are often more daunting than the reality we face. It might take some time to discover what approach resonates with you, but the insights and tranquility you'll gain will be well worth it. It's a journey of not just better sleep but profound self-discovery.

Evening Sleep Journal

Incorporate this journal into your evening wind-down routine.

Today's Date: _____

Write down the time/description for each item.

Caffeine	
Supplements	
Medications	
Exercise	
Evening Meal	
Snacks	
Beverages	
Alcohol	
Naps	

My Sleepiness Level Today (Low / Medium / High)

My Stress Level Today (Low / Medium / High)

Can you make any connections to activities that impacted sleep?

DAY 19

Breath work for Stress Reduction

Let's talk about a secret sleep weapon that's always within your reach – your breath. Tuning into your breath is an incredibly effective way to quiet a restless mind and soothe a tense body, guiding you into a relaxed state that's perfect for drifting off to sleep. But it's not just at night when breath work comes into its own. I've also found it to be a lifeline during the day, helping to reduce stress, sharpen focus, and reboot my calm at a moment's notice.

For years, I've been practicing breathwork techniques, both for sleep and during the chaotic hours of my waking life. I've found it so beneficial that I even keep a sticky note on my car dashboard that says 'Breathe.' It's a gentle nudge to take a moment, inhale, exhale, and regain my center when I find myself at a red light or when traffic is testing my patience. Complete your Morning Sleep Journal, and then let me share some of the breathing techniques that have become my go-to relaxation tools:

Morning Sleep Journal

Complete this each morning to see the impact on your daily sleep!

Today's Date: _____   Bedtime Last Night: _____

How well did you fall asleep?

___ Easily   ___ It took a while   ___ It was difficult

Describe what it was like falling asleep:

Did you wake up and struggle to fall back asleep?

___ Not at all   ___ Once or twice   ___ Multiple times

Describe your experience:

Wake-Up Time: _____   Total Hours of Sleep _____

How did you feel after waking up?

___ Refreshed   ___ Just okay   ___ Tired

Notes:

Box Breathing (4-4-4-4)

This technique helps to calm the mind and regulate the breath and is often used by military personnel and first responders to manage stress.

- Inhale for 4 seconds
- Hold your breath for 4 seconds
- Exhale (slowly) for 4 seconds
- Hold the breath again for 4 seconds
- Repeat the cycle for a few minutes or until you feel relaxed

4-7-8 Breathing

This technique, also known as the "relaxing breath," is designed to act as a natural tranquilizer for the nervous system, promoting relaxation and reducing anxiety.

- Inhale for 4 seconds
- Hold the breath for 7 seconds
- Exhale for 8 seconds
- Repeat the cycle for 4 breaths or until feeling relaxed

Diaphragmatic Breathing (Belly Breathing)

This technique encourages full oxygen exchange and helps to strengthen the diaphragm, leading to deeper, more efficient breathing and relaxation.

- Place one hand on the chest and the other on the abdomen
- Take a slow, deep breath through the nose, allowing the abdomen to rise
- Exhale slowly through the mouth or nose, allowing the abdomen to fall
- Repeat the cycle for a few minutes or until you feel relaxed

Alternate Nostril Breathing (Nadi Shodhana)

This technique, commonly practiced in yoga, helps to balance the left and right sides of the brain and promotes mental clarity and relaxation.

- Use the right thumb to close the right nostril
- Inhale through the left nostril
- Close the left nostril with the right ring finger, open the right nostril, and exhale
- Inhale through the right nostril, close it, open the left nostril, and exhale
- Repeat the cycle for a few minutes or until feeling relaxed

Final Notes on Breathing

Remember to practice these breathing techniques in a comfortable, quiet environment. They can be easily incorporated throughout the day and into your bedtime routine to help promote relaxation and improve sleep quality.

Now it is time to complete your Evening Sleep Journal before getting into a good night's sleep.

Evening Sleep Journal

Incorporate this journal into your evening wind-down routine.

Today's Date: _____

Write down the time/description for each item.

Caffeine	
Supplements	
Medications	
Exercise	
Evening Meal	
Snacks	
Beverages	
Alcohol	
Naps	

My Sleepiness Level Today (Low / Medium / High)

My Stress Level Today (Low / Medium / High)

Can you make any connections to activities that impacted sleep?

DAY 20

Become a Zen Master

For the past decade, my journey with meditation has been a dance - sometimes fluid, sometimes a bit clumsy. Just as I get into a rhythm, life, with its impeccable timing, steps in and diverts my course. Yet, no matter how long the breaks, I always find myself drawn back to the quiet serenity it provides, especially for my sleep.

Meditation is akin to training for the mind. It's a powerful tool that not only helps mitigate stress but also reigns in my habitually busy mind, steering it away from incessant rumination. And let me tell you, the difference it makes to a good night's sleep is remarkable.

Before we get started with the many types of meditation available, finish your Morning Sleep Journal.

Morning Sleep Journal

Complete this each morning to see the impact on your daily sleep!

Today's Date: _____   Bedtime Last Night: _____

How well did you fall asleep?

___ Easily   ____ It took a while   ____ It was difficult

Describe what it was like falling asleep:

Did you wake up and struggle to fall back asleep?

___ Not at all   ____ Once or twice   ____ Multiple times

Describe your experience:

Wake-Up Time: _____   Total Hours of Sleep _____

How did you feel after waking up?

___ Refreshed   ____ Just okay   ____ Tired

Notes:

What Meditation Is (and Isn't)

Meditation has long been recognized as a powerful tool to calm the mind and reduce negative thoughts. Scientific research has demonstrated the mechanisms behind these effects, revealing that meditation can alter brainwave patterns and neural connections. When we meditate, our brainwaves shift from high-frequency beta waves, associated with active thinking and worry, to lower-frequency alpha and theta waves, which are linked to relaxation and mental clarity.

Furthermore, regular meditation practice has strengthened the prefrontal and anterior cortex, brain regions responsible for self-awareness, emotional regulation, and cognitive control. This increased neural resilience allows us to manage stress better and break free from negative thought patterns.

By incorporating meditation into your nightly routine, you can cultivate a more balanced and peaceful state of mind, promoting improved mental well-being and sleep quality.

There are several types of meditation that are particularly beneficial for sleep.

Body Scan Meditation

Promote deep relaxation by cultivating awareness of the body and releasing tension.

- Lie down or sit comfortably with your eyes closed.
- Bring attention to each body part, starting with the toes and moving up to the head.
- Observe any sensations, tension, or discomfort in each area and release tension with each exhale.

Loving-Kindness Meditation (Metta)

Foster positive emotions, reduce negative thoughts, and cultivate compassion, leading to a more restful sleep.

- Sit or lie down comfortably with your eyes closed.
- Silently repeat phrases such as "May I be happy, may I be healthy, may I be safe, may I be at ease" to cultivate feelings of love and kindness towards oneself.
- Gradually extend these sentiments to loved ones, acquaintances, and even those with whom you have difficulties.

Guided Imagery Meditation

Calm the mind by focusing on soothing, positive images, and can be particularly helpful for those with an overactive imagination or racing thoughts.

- Lie down or sit comfortably with your eyes closed.
- Listen to a guided meditation or visualize a peaceful, calming scene in your mind, such as a beach, forest, or meadow.
- Allow the mind to explore the scene, engaging all the senses, and let the imagery promote relaxation and tranquility.

Mindfulness Meditation

Cultivate present-moment awareness and encourage the mind to let go of worries or concerns, promoting relaxation and improved sleep quality.

- Lie down or sit comfortably with your eyes closed.
- Focus on the natural rhythm of your breath, observing each inhale and exhale without judgment.
- If the mind wanders, gently bring it back to the breath.

Yoga Nidra (Yogic Sleep)

This practice is designed to induce a state of deep relaxation while remaining conscious and can be an effective way to unwind and prepare the body and mind for sleep.

- Lie down comfortably with your eyes closed.
- Listen to a guided yoga nidra meditation or follow a script focusing on deep relaxation and the transition between waking and sleeping.
- Experiment with these different meditation techniques to find the one that works best for you. Incorporating meditation into your bedtime routine can create a sense of calm and relaxation that will help improve your sleep quality and overall well-being.

Practice, Practice, Practice

Are you ready to become a Zen Master? Start practicing these techniques, and you will be well on your way.

For now, complete your Evening Sleep Journal.

Evening Sleep Journal

Incorporate this journal into your evening wind-down routine.

Today's Date: _____

Write down the time/description for each item.

Caffeine	
Supplements	
Medications	
Exercise	
Evening Meal	
Snacks	
Beverages	
Alcohol	
Naps	

My Sleepiness Level Today (Low / Medium / High)

My Stress Level Today (Low / Medium / High)

Can you make any connections to activities that impacted sleep?

DAY 21

We're wrapping up Week 3, and it's been all about mastering your mind for better sleep.

Did the techniques of reframing, meditation, and breath work help in settling down before bed? How effective were the 'To-do' and 'Worry lists' in helping you clear your thoughts?

It's essential to remember that different strategies resonate with different people. Take note of what's working for you and stick with it. The real benefits come with consistency.

As we head into Week 4, we're going to shift gears. We'll dive into your 'Sleep Toolbox' and introduce practical tools to enhance your sleep routines and quality.

Let's keep pushing forward on this sleep journey!

Today, all you need to do is complete your Morning and Evening Journal.

Morning Sleep Journal

Complete this each morning to see the impact on your daily sleep!

Today's Date: _____   Bedtime Last Night: _____

How well did you fall asleep?

___ Easily   ____ It took a while   ____ It was difficult

Describe what it was like falling asleep:

Did you wake up and struggle to fall back asleep?

___ Not at all   ____ Once or twice   ____ Multiple times

Describe your experience:

Wake-Up Time: _____   Total Hours of Sleep _____

How did you feel after waking up?

___ Refreshed   ____ Just okay   ____ Tired

Notes:

Evening Sleep Journal

Incorporate this journal into your evening wind-down routine.

Today's Date: _____

Write down the time/description for each item.

Caffeine	
Supplements	
Medications	
Exercise	
Evening Meal	
Snacks	
Beverages	
Alcohol	
Naps	

My Sleepiness Level Today (Low / Medium / High)

My Stress Level Today (Low / Medium / High)

Can you make any connections to activities that impacted sleep?

WEEK 4

Your Sleep Toolbox

Welcome to Week 4, where we'll dive into the world of sleep aids, exploring the gadgets, apps, and sleep enhancers that can turn the dream of a perfect night's sleep into a reality! This week, we highlight tools and technologies that can complement the strategies we've already discussed and add an extra layer of support to your sleep-improvement journey.

DAY 22

Sleep Wearables and Apps

From innovative devices that monitor and optimize your sleep environment to smart apps that guide you through relaxing meditations, today we'll explore a variety of tools you can add to your personal sleep toolbox.

But first, complete your Morning Sleep Journal.

Morning Sleep Journal

Complete this each morning to see the impact on your daily sleep!

Today's Date: _____   Bedtime Last Night: _____

How well did you fall asleep?

___ Easily   ____ It took a while   ____ It was difficult

Describe what it was like falling asleep:

Did you wake up and struggle to fall back asleep?

___ Not at all   ____ Once or twice   ____ Multiple times

Describe your experience:

Wake-Up Time: _____   Total Hours of Sleep _____

How did you feel after waking up?

___ Refreshed   ____ Just okay   ____ Tired

Notes:

Sleep Wearables

I've always been a bit of a tracker-junkie, finding joy in keeping tabs on everything from my nutrition, heart rate, and daily steps to even how many consecutive days I've been meditating. So, you can imagine my excitement when sleep trackers started to hit the scene.

Although investing in a sleep tracker isn't necessary for everyone looking to improve their sleep, it can be a fun way to provide deeper insight into your sleep patterns. Here is a list of popular ones currently on the market.

Oura Ring

This is not your average piece of jewelry. Oura Ring is a sleek, comfortable ring that tracks your sleep and gives you detailed reports about your sleep stages, heart rate, and more. It's discreet, stylish, and packed with cutting-edge tech. It's like having a sleep scientist right on your finger.

I have been wearing an Oura Ring for over a year, which has helped me find connections between my daily lifestyle habits and my sleep quality. For instance, when I eat a late meal or drink alcohol in the evening, I can see how my deep sleep and REM sleep are negatively impacted. It is also comfortable to sleep with.

Sleep and Meditation Apps

Sleep and Meditation Apps are another great resource for insomniacs. These apps typically offer various features such as guided meditation, sleep tracking, soothing sounds, bedtime stories, and breathing exercises. Let's take a look at a few popular ones.

Calm

This popular app (my personal favorite) offers guided meditations, sleep stories, breathing programs, and relaxing music. A unique feature is its selection of nature sounds and celebrity-narrated sleep stories.

Headspace

A user-friendly app that provides an array of guided meditations. It includes a specific section for sleep, featuring meditations, soundscapes, and sleep casts (stories) designed to create the right conditions for healthy, restful sleep.

10% Happier

Aimed at "fidgety skeptics," this app features a variety of meditation courses, including ones specifically for sleep and stress. Some of the "teachers" are celebrities or experienced monks. It also includes bedtime stories and soundscapes.

Apple Watch

Apple Watch has many great features, including tracking your sleep. With the Sleep app on Apple Watch, you can set and achieve your sleep goals, giving you a detailed analysis of your sleep patterns. Plus, it's an Apple product, so you know you're getting a top-notch piece of technology.

Fitbit

Fitbit has been a big name in the fitness-tracking world for a while, but did you know it also tracks your sleep? It measures your sleep stages, tracks your heart rate, and even has a silent alarm to wake you gently. It's like having a personal trainer and a sleep coach all in one device!

Garmin

Known for its GPS technology, Garmin also offers a range of fitness wearables that provide sleep-tracking features. Devices like the Garmin Vivosmart 4 track sleep stages and measure your body's oxygen levels during sleep, a feature not commonly found in other wearables.

There's a whole range of sleep-tracking wearables out there, each with its own unique features. Remember, the best one for you depends on your personal needs and preferences. So, do your research, and pick the one that suits you best.

Insight Timer

With more than 70,000 free guided meditations, music tracks, talks, and courses, Insight Timer offers many options for all experience levels. It has an extensive library of sleep, relaxation, and stress relief tracks.

White Noise Lite

Provides ambient sounds of the environment to help you relax or sleep. This app is highly recommended for blocking distractions, traveling, calming babies, and even masking tinnitus.

Sleep Score

This app tracks your sleep with nothing but your smartphone itself; no separate devices are needed. It provides a detailed analysis of your sleep stages and offers personalized advice to improve sleep quality.

Many of these apps have free trials. Experiment with a few to find one that works for you.

You know what is next - time for your Evening Sleep Journal!

Evening Sleep Journal

Incorporate this journal into your evening wind-down routine.

Today's Date: _____

Write down the time/description for each item.

Caffeine	
Supplements	
Medications	
Exercise	
Evening Meal	
Snacks	
Beverages	
Alcohol	
Naps	

My Sleepiness Level Today (Low / Medium / High)

My Stress Level Today (Low / Medium / High)

Can you make any connections to activities that impacted sleep?

DAY 23

Ambient Noise

Could noise actually promote better sleep? Absolutely! But the catch is, it has to be the right kind of noise. While unexpected loud noises can jolt you awake, consistent, ambient sounds can mask external interruptions, lulling your brain into a peaceful slumber. Today, we'll explore the science and benefits of noise enhancing your sleep experience.

First, complete your Morning Sleep Journal. Then, we will dive in on the science of noise.

Morning Sleep Journal

Complete this each morning to see the impact on your daily sleep!

Today's Date: _____   Bedtime Last Night: _____

How well did you fall asleep?

___ Easily   ___ It took a while   ___ It was difficult

Describe what it was like falling asleep:

Did you wake up and struggle to fall back asleep?

___ Not at all   ___ Once or twice   ___ Multiple times

Describe your experience:

Wake-Up Time: _____   Total Hours of Sleep _____

How did you feel after waking up?

___ Refreshed   ___ Just okay   ___ Tired

Notes:

White Noise

One form of noise that can help you sleep is white noise. So, what is white noise? Well, in the simplest terms, it's a special type of sound signal that's used to mask background noises.

"But how does it help me sleep?" you might ask. When it's quiet, your brain sometimes starts to search for sounds, and that can keep you awake. Even small, sudden noises like a car passing by or a door closing can jolt you awake. That's where white noise comes in. It creates a constant, soothing backdrop of sound, so those little noises aren't as noticeable.

White noise can be particularly helpful if you live in a noisy environment, have a partner who snores, or find it hard to fall asleep because of a racing mind. There are plenty of white noise machines available, or even apps that you can download on your phone, that offer a variety of sounds - from gentle rainfall to the whir of a fan (I love cranking up my ceiling fan).

Believe it or not, there are other "colored" noises out there that are known to help with sleep.

Brown Noise

Known to be deeper than white noise, brown noise can be more effective than white noise for some people.

Pink Noise

Somewhere between white noise and brown noise, pink noise sounds like steady rain or rustling leaves. Sleep studies have shown a link to improved memory, sleep, and relaxation. Like with white noise, you can find apps that offer an array of noises, such as the app Simply Noise. Experiment with different options. You might find your ticket to Dreamland!

Binaural Beats

Imagine you're listening to two different tunes, one in each ear, and your brain creates a whole new tune from the difference between them. This new tune is known as a 'binaural beat.'

Why does this matter for sleep? Our brains have different types of 'waves' that match how we feel. For instance, our brain has slow, calming waves when we're relaxed. When we're alert, our brain has fast, active waves.

Now, this is where binaural beats come in. Playing two different sounds can trick our brain into making those slow, calming waves that help us feel relaxed and sleepy.

Some people find that listening to binaural beats as part of their bedtime routine helps them fall asleep faster and sleep deeper. I have found them helpful to lull me back to sleep when I wake up in the middle of the night, and my brain goes into overdrive. I focus on the sounds and let the beats do the rest. It has really helped me to fall back to sleep.

To experience the benefits of binaural beats for yourself, consider the following tips:

• Choose high-quality binaural beat recordings designed specifically for sleep. Look for recordings in the delta and theta frequency ranges. You can find a great selection of Binaural Beats on YouTube and the App/Google Play Store. In addition, many sleep apps offer a binaural beats option.

• Use headphones or earbuds for the best results, as they allow each ear to receive a separate frequency.

• Listen to binaural beats as part of your bedtime routine to signal to your brain that it's time to wind down and prepare for sleep.

• Experiment with different binaural beat frequencies and durations to find what works best for you.

It's important to note that binaural beats are not a one-size-fits-all solution, and individual experiences may vary. However, incorporating binaural beats into your sleep routine may help improve your sleep quality and provide a natural, non-pharmacological approach to better rest.

Give noise a try!

But first, go ahead and fill out your Evening Sleep Journal for today.

Evening Sleep Journal

Incorporate this journal into your evening wind-down routine.

Today's Date: _____

Write down the time/description for each item.

Caffeine	
Supplements	
Medications	
Exercise	
Evening Meal	
Snacks	
Beverages	
Alcohol	
Naps	

My Sleepiness Level Today (Low / Medium / High)

My Stress Level Today (Low / Medium / High)

Can you make any connections to activities that impacted sleep?

DAY 24

Blue Blocking Glasses

Blue-blocking glasses have been my sleep savior. I have worn them consistently for the last ten years (much to my husband's dismay). I put them on at around 9:00 every night while watching TV or reading my Nook. I honestly feel myself getting sleepy as soon as I put them on.

Blue-blocking glasses work by filtering out sleep-stealing blue light, thus helping your body to produce the melatonin you need to get your shut-eye. By donning a pair of these glasses in the evening, you're helping your body maintain its natural sleep rhythm.

You can find a variety of blue-blocking glasses online. But not all blue blockers are created equal.

I will share what to look for, but first, complete your Morning Sleep Journal.

Morning Sleep Journal

Complete this each morning to see the impact on your daily sleep!

Today's Date: _____   Bedtime Last Night: _____

How well did you fall asleep?

___ Easily   ____ It took a while   ____ It was difficult

Describe what it was like falling asleep:

Did you wake up and struggle to fall back asleep?

___ Not at all   ____ Once or twice   ____ Multiple times

Describe your experience:

Wake-Up Time: _____   Total Hours of Sleep _____

How did you feel after waking up?

___ Refreshed   ____ Just okay   ____ Tired

Notes:

Percentage of Blue Light Blocked

These glasses aren't just about looking cool - they have a job to do! Look for ones that tell you the percentage of blue light they block - the more, the merrier.

Fit and Coverage

Like a trendy pair of sunglasses, your blue light-blocking glasses must fit snugly and cover your eyes well. If light sneaks in from the sides, those glasses aren't doing their full job.

Specific Wavelengths Blocked

Blue light comes in different wavelengths, from about 380 to 500 nm. The wavelengths that are messing with your sleep are typically in the 460-480 nm range. Glasses focusing on this range might be your best bet for better sleep.

Comfort and Style

Finally, let's be real - you're going to wear these glasses a lot, so they've got to feel good and look good. The perfect balance of comfort and style makes the whole experience much more enjoyable.

If you struggle to fall asleep after a late-night Netflix binge or hours spent scrolling through social media, blue light-blocking glasses are what you need to add to your toolbox.

Evening Sleep Journal

Incorporate this journal into your evening wind-down routine.

Today's Date: _____

Write down the time/description for each item.

Caffeine	
Supplements	
Medications	
Exercise	
Evening Meal	
Snacks	
Beverages	
Alcohol	
Naps	

My Sleepiness Level Today (Low / Medium / High)

My Stress Level Today (Low / Medium / High)

Can you make any connections to activities that impacted sleep?

DAY 25

Weighted Blankets

Are you looking for a warm hug, but there's no one around to give it to you? Well, a weighted blanket might be the comforting companion you need.

Weighted blankets offer a form of touch pressure called 'deep pressure stimulation,' which feels like a firm hug, a massage, or swaddling. But what does this have to do with sleep, you ask?

We will answer that question right after you complete your Morning Sleep Journal.

Morning Sleep Journal

Complete this each morning to see the impact on your daily sleep!

Today's Date: _____   Bedtime Last Night: _____

How well did you fall asleep?

___ Easily   ____ It took a while   ____ It was difficult

Describe what it was like falling asleep:

Did you wake up and struggle to fall back asleep?

___ Not at all   ____ Once or twice   ____ Multiple times

Describe your experience:

Wake-Up Time: _____   Total Hours of Sleep _____

How did you feel after waking up?

___ Refreshed   ____ Just okay   ____ Tired

Notes:

Why Weighted Blankets Work

The answer lies in our biology. This deep-pressure stimulation has been shown to increase the release of a hormone called serotonin, a mood-lifting hormone that our body uses to make – you guessed it – melatonin!

Not only that, but the comforting pressure can also help reduce activity in the nervous system, calming an overactive mind and leading to a sense of relaxation. This can be particularly beneficial if you tend to toss and turn with thoughts whirling like a tornado in your mind.

I love my weighted blanket. So much so that I recently purchased a weighted eye mask! A weighted eye mask works on the same principle. It provides a soothing pressure across your eyes and forehead, which can help to relieve tension and aid in relaxation. It's like a do-not-disturb sign for your brain!

When considering a weighted blanket, there are a few key things to consider.

Weight

The general recommendation is to choose a blanket that's about 10% of your body weight. For instance, if you weigh 150 pounds, a 15-pound blanket would be appropriate. However, personal preference plays a role, so you might prefer something lighter or heavier.

Size

Weighted blankets come in various sizes. Rather than fitting your bed, they're designed to fit the user. Make sure it covers you comfortably without hanging too much over the sides of the bed, which can pull the blanket off.

Material

They can be made from various fabrics, including cotton, flannel, Minky, and bamboo. Choose a fabric based on your personal preference for warmth and texture. Some people may prefer a breathable cotton for warmer climates, while others might want the plush feel of Minky.

Filling

The weight in these blankets comes from materials such as plastic pellets, glass beads, or even steel shots. Glass beads are generally smoother and denser than plastic pellets, providing a finer, more contoured feel.

Construction

Look for a blanket with a baffle-box or quilted construction, which helps ensure the weight is evenly distributed, and the filler doesn't shift.

Washability

Some weighted blankets are machine washable, while others have a removable cover for easier cleaning. Consider how often you'll want to wash it and your capacity to handle its bulk in your washer and dryer.

Temperature Regulation

If you tend to get hot while sleeping, look for weighted blankets that have cooling technologies or breathable fabrics to avoid overheating.

Price

Weighted blankets can range significantly in price. While cost often correlates with quality, there are plenty of reasonably priced options that are also well-made.

If you're longing for a warm, comforting hug that can help you drift off into the land of dreams, a weighted blanket might be worth considering. You can find a variety of weighted blankets online. Pick the weight and material that suits your fancy. Pair it with a weighted eye mask, and you've got yourself a sleep-inducing superhero duo!

Evening Sleep Journal

Incorporate this journal into your evening wind-down routine.

Today's Date: _____

Write down the time/description for each item.

Caffeine	
Supplements	
Medications	
Exercise	
Evening Meal	
Snacks	
Beverages	
Alcohol	
Naps	

My Sleepiness Level Today (Low / Medium / High)

My Stress Level Today (Low / Medium / High)

Can you make any connections to activities that impacted sleep?

DAY 26

Relax with Aromatherapy

Aromatherapy, the art of using essential oils for wellness, can be a game-changer when it comes to sleep. Essential oils use the super-concentrated, fragrant essences of plants and have been used for centuries to promote relaxation and well-being.

Let's chat about a few superstar oils for sleep right after you complete your Morning Sleep Journal.

Morning Sleep Journal

Complete this each morning to see the impact on your daily sleep!

Today's Date: _____   Bedtime Last Night: _____

How well did you fall asleep?

___ Easily   ___ It took a while   ___ It was difficult

Describe what it was like falling asleep:

Did you wake up and struggle to fall back asleep?

___ Not at all   ___ Once or twice   ___ Multiple times

Describe your experience:

Wake-Up Time: _____   Total Hours of Sleep _____

How did you feel after waking up?

___ Refreshed   ___ Just okay   ___ Tired

Notes:

Lavender

This one's the big kahuna of sleep-friendly scents. Lavender is well-loved for its calming, relaxing properties. A few drops in your diffuser, and you'll feel like you're drifting off in a peaceful meadow. Personally, I like to add lavender oil to my Epsom salt bath. You can also find lavender-scented lotions and pillow sprays.

Chamomile

You've probably had chamomile tea, but have you tried chamomile essential oil? It's a gentle, comforting scent, perfect for easing the mind before bedtime. You can add a few drops to your diffuser. Dilute it with a carrier oil and apply it to pulse points for a gentle, calming effect. Or breathe in the scent directly by adding a drop or two to a cloth or tissue.

Bergamot

Unlike most citrus oils that are stimulating, bergamot is calming. It can help reduce anxiety and promote relaxation. The unique citrusy yet calming aroma of bergamot can fill your room when used in a diffuser. As with the others, always dilute bergamot oil with a carrier oil before applying to the skin, especially since it can be photosensitive (it can increase the risk of sunburn).

Before You Get Started...

Here are a couple of important tips to keep in mind for safety and maximum efficacy.

Less is more.

A few drops are usually all you need for an effective aroma.

Safety first!

Essential oils are powerful stuff. Never apply them directly to your skin. Instead, dilute them in a carrier oil or use an aromatherapy diffuser. Remember, when introducing a new essential oil to your routine, it's always a good idea to do a patch test to ensure you don't have an allergic reaction. Always consult with a professional if you're pregnant, nursing, or have a medical condition before using essential oils.

Experiment! Everyone's nose is different. What smells heavenly to one person might be too strong for another. So, try out a few oils to see what you enjoy most.

Evening Sleep Journal

Incorporate this journal into your evening wind-down routine.

Today's Date: _____

Write down the time/description for each item.

Caffeine	
Supplements	
Medications	
Exercise	
Evening Meal	
Snacks	
Beverages	
Alcohol	
Naps	

My Sleepiness Level Today (Low / Medium / High)

My Stress Level Today (Low / Medium / High)

Can you make any connections to activities that impacted sleep?

DAY 27

Supplements for Sleep

There are a variety of supplements on the market that have been shown to improve the onset, duration, and quality of sleep. However, this is not a one-size-fits-all formula. What works for your coworker or a TikTok influencer may not work for you.

Another consideration is that the FDA does not regulate supplements, so you do not always know if what is stated on the label is in the pill.

Having said all of that, here's a list of some supplements associated with improved sleep. (Right after your Morning Sleep Journal, of course.)

Morning Sleep Journal

Complete this each morning to see the impact on your daily sleep!

Today's Date: _____   Bedtime Last Night: _____

How well did you fall asleep?

___ Easily   ___ It took a while   ___ It was difficult

Describe what it was like falling asleep:

Did you wake up and struggle to fall back asleep?

___ Not at all   ___ Once or twice   ___ Multiple times

Describe your experience:

Wake-Up Time: _____   Total Hours of Sleep _____

How did you feel after waking up?

___ Refreshed   ___ Just okay   ___ Tired

Notes:

Melatonin

As we have already discussed, melatonin is the hormone that is secreted from our brain's pineal gland to help regulate sleep-wake cycles. Ideally, your circadian rhythms are in sync, and you are secreting your own melatonin like a champ. But if that is not yet the case, temporary supplementation may help. Also, according to the Sleep Foundation, our melatonin production decreases as we age. If you feel that may be the case, consult your doctor regarding long-term use.

Melatonin comes in various doses and is available as a pill, liquid, chewable, and sublingual supplement. More is not always better. You can start with the lowest dose possible (a pill cutter can be useful in this situation). Also, some people say that melatonin helps them to fall asleep initially, but it does not help with sleep duration. This was the case for me until I began using "extended-release" melatonin.

While melatonin can be found in some foods like cherries, tomatoes, and walnuts, the amount is usually too small to impact sleep significantly. You should also consult your doctor before using melatonin, especially if you are taking blood thinners, anticoagulants, anticonvulsants, or medications for diabetes.

Valerian Root

Valerian root is an herbal supplement commonly used for insomnia and anxiety. It is usually available in capsule, tablet, and liquid extract forms. You will also find it in teas meant for sleep enhancement, as well as over-the-counter sleep formulas. Valerian root can interact with certain medications, such as sedatives, anesthetics, and medications for anxiety or depression, so it's essential to consult with your healthcare provider before using it.

Chamomile

Chamomile is an herb known for its calming effects and is often used as a sleep aid. It is typically consumed as a tea, but can also be found in capsule and liquid extract forms. Chamomile can interact with blood thinners, sedatives, and medications for anxiety or depression, so consult your healthcare provider before using it.

Lavender

Lavender is an herb known for its calming and sleep-promoting properties. Lavender supplements are available as capsules, essential oils, and pillow sprays. Be cautious when using lavender in combination with sedatives, as it can increase their effects.

Magnesium

Magnesium is a mineral that is responsible for more than 300 chemical reactions in the body. Muscles need this mineral to contract; nerves need it to send and receive messages. It keeps your heart beating steadily and your immune system strong. Magnesium is also believed to play a role in muscle relaxation and supports healthy sleep patterns.

Magnesium supplements come in various forms; however, magnesium glycinate or magnesium threonate is often recommended for sleep due to its high bioavailability and calming effect on the nervous system.

Magnesium can also be found in foods like spinach, pumpkin seeds, almonds, and avocados. Be cautious when using magnesium supplements if you are taking medications for osteoporosis, heart conditions, or antibiotics, as it can interact with these drugs.

According to the National Institute of Health, an adult woman's recommended daily magnesium intake is between 300 and 320 milligrams (mg), and 400 to 420 mg for an adult man.

L-theanine

L-theanine is an amino acid found in green tea. According to neuroscientist and sleep specialist Dr. Andrew Huberman, taking a supplement of L-theanine before bedtime will get your brain to attempt to reach REM as much as possible. This means you can fall asleep faster and spend more time dreaming.

L-theanine is an extract from green tea. Studies have shown that L-theanine may help a person fall asleep faster and spend more time in bed dreaming, as well as give individuals a more restful sleep.

Apigenin

Apigenin is a natural flavonoid found in plants like chamomile and parsley. It has been shown to have calming and sleep-promoting effects. It also helps to calm a racing mind (I know this firsthand).

Apigenin is available as a supplement in capsule form and can also be found in foods like celery, oranges, and grapefruit. There is limited information on potential drug interactions with apigenin, so consult your healthcare provider before using it, especially if you are taking other medications.

Adaptogens

Adaptogens are a unique class of healing plants that can help enhance the body's ability to resist stress. They are named for their adaptive properties, which enable them to respond to your body's needs. Adaptogens such as ashwagandha, Holy Basil (Tulsi), and Rhodiola rosea can be particularly beneficial for sleep. These plants have been used for centuries in traditional medicine for their calming and restorative effects. They work by helping to balance your body's adrenal system, which regulates your body's hormonal response to stress. This can result in improved sleep quality, reduced stress levels, and a general feeling of calm and well-being.

Cannabidiol (CBD)

CBD has gained traction in recent years for its potential benefits on sleep. Unlike THC (the psychoactive compound found in marijuana), CBD doesn't make you "high," but it is believed to impact sleep by interacting with a network of receptors, proteins, and other chemicals in the brain that influence all sorts of things, including anxiety and sleep-wake cycles.

Some people find that taking a CBD supplement can help them feel more relaxed and calmer before bedtime, paving the way for a more restful night's sleep. But remember, research is still in its infancy, and it's crucial to talk to a healthcare provider before starting any new supplement routine, including CBD. Also, look for high-quality, third-party-tested products to ensure you get what's on the label.

Remember to always check with your healthcare provider before starting any supplements. This is especially important if you have a medical condition or take prescription medications.

Prescription Sleep Medications

This program aims to help you get to the underlying cause of your insomnia, so you do not have to resort to prescription sleep aids. But for those of you who are considering or currently taking sleep prescriptions, here's what you need to know.

Prescription sleep medications can provide short-term relief for insomnia and other sleep disorders, but are not without risks. Understanding the pros and cons of these medications is essential for making informed decisions about your sleep health.

Pros to Sleep Medication

Short-term relief: Sleep medications can temporarily relieve individuals struggling with chronic insomnia or other sleep disorders, helping them fall asleep faster and stay asleep longer.

Enhanced sleep quality: For those with severe sleep issues, prescription sleep aids can improve overall sleep quality, leading to increased daytime alertness and better overall functioning.

Guided usage: When prescribed by a doctor, sleep medications are typically accompanied by professional guidance and monitoring, ensuring safe and appropriate usage.

Cons to Sleep Medication

Potential side effects: Prescription sleep aids can cause various side effects, including dizziness, daytime drowsiness, headaches, and gastrointestinal issues. In some cases, these medications can also lead to more severe side effects such as sleepwalking, sleep-related eating disorders, and memory problems.

Risk of dependency: Long-term use of sleep medications can result in physical or psychological dependence, making it challenging to stop using them without experiencing withdrawal symptoms or rebound insomnia.

Interaction with other medications: Sleep medications can interact with other drugs, potentially causing dangerous side effects or reducing the effectiveness of either medication.

Masking underlying issues: Relying on sleep medications without addressing the root cause of sleep issues can be a temporary solution, merely masking the real problem rather than resolving it.

Please work with your physician if you are contemplating prescription sleep medications. It is imperative to know how they may interact with other medications or supplements you are currently taking. You will also want to devise a tapering-off strategy so they do not become a long-term crutch.

Evening Sleep Journal

Incorporate this journal into your evening wind-down routine.

Today's Date: _____

Write down the time/description for each item.

Caffeine	
Supplements	
Medications	
Exercise	
Evening Meal	
Snacks	
Beverages	
Alcohol	
Naps	

My Sleepiness Level Today (Low / Medium / High)

My Stress Level Today (Low / Medium / High)

Can you make any connections to activities that impacted sleep?

DAY 28

Week 4 Check-In

Hello, fellow sleep warriors! We're now closing off an exciting week of exploring your sleep toolbox. As we took a more tangible approach to improving sleep, it was a time for you to be hands-on and experimental. How did that go for you?

Did you find any gadgets, apps, or sleep enhancers that seem to help your sleep patterns? Or perhaps you're still exploring and trying to find the perfect tool that fits your needs. Remember, it's all about finding what works best for you and your unique sleep rhythm.

This week, I encourage you to play the role of an intrepid sleep explorer: investigate, test out, and adopt one or more sleep tools into your nightly routine. Whether it's a sleep-promoting app, a dreamy, weighted blanket, or a soothing sound machine, find the tool or tools that resonate with you most. Remember, this is your journey to better sleep, and you get to customize it to your liking!

Morning Sleep Journal

Complete this each morning to see the impact on your daily sleep!

Today's Date: _____   Bedtime Last Night: _____

How well did you fall asleep?

___ Easily   ___ It took a while   ___ It was difficult

Describe what it was like falling asleep:

Did you wake up and struggle to fall back asleep?

___ Not at all   ___ Once or twice   ___ Multiple times

Describe your experience:

Wake-Up Time: _____   Total Hours of Sleep _____

How did you feel after waking up?

___ Refreshed   ___ Just okay   ___ Tired

Notes:

In addition to this adventurous quest, we'll also be continuing with our journaling exercises. Yes, it's still on the menu, but for good reasons! The reflective practice is essential in helping you uncover your sleep patterns, understand your stressors, and keep track of your progress. Let's keep up the good work! Continue to pour out your thoughts, worries, and achievements, letting your journal serve as your guide and confidante on this sleep-transforming journey.

Now, as we transition into the home stretch, this next phase is all about peeling back the layers and looking beneath the surface. We'll explore potential areas that might be impacting your sleep, such as hormones, blood sugar, and hydration, and even explore the possibility of underlying sleep disorders. So, let's gear up and get ready to dig deeper!

Morning Sleep Journal

Complete this each morning to see the impact on your daily sleep!

Today's Date: _____   Bedtime Last Night: _____

How well did you fall asleep?

___ Easily   ____ It took a while   ____ It was difficult

Describe what it was like falling asleep:

Did you wake up and struggle to fall back asleep?

___ Not at all   ____ Once or twice   ____ Multiple times

Describe your experience:

Wake-Up Time: _____   Total Hours of Sleep _____

How did you feel after waking up?

___ Refreshed   ____ Just okay   ____ Tired

Notes:

Evening Sleep Journal

Incorporate this journal into your evening wind-down routine.

Today's Date: _____

Write down the time/description for each item.

Caffeine	
Supplements	
Medications	
Exercise	
Evening Meal	
Snacks	
Beverages	
Alcohol	
Naps	

My Sleepiness Level Today (Low / Medium / High)

My Stress Level Today (Low / Medium / High)

Can you make any connections to activities that impacted sleep?

WEEK 5

Digging Deeper

Welcome to Week 5! Until now, we've explored the essentials of sleep hygiene, the importance of routine, the role of daily activities in sleep quality, calming your mind chatter, and great tools to enhance your sleep. You've started unraveling the mystery of your insomnia, but if you're still struggling, don't despair!

This week, we're digging deeper. We're diving into the undercurrents that may be subtly but significantly disrupting your sleep: factors like hormonal imbalances, blood sugar irregularities, dehydration, nocturia, food sensitivities, and potential sleep disorders. These complex elements often stay hidden in the shadows, yet their influence on your sleep is profound. Understanding and addressing these elements can be the key to unlocking the restful night's sleep you've been yearning for.

So, let's embark on this deeper journey and continue our quest to conquer your insomnia! Let's explore potential culprits, starting with blood sugar regulation.

DAY 29

Blood Sugar Imbalances

Are you riding the blood sugar roller coaster? If your blood sugar is out of whack, not only will it impact your energy, moods, weight and set you on a path to diabetes, it can seriously screw up your sleep.

After you complete your Morning Sleep Journal, I will give you all the details!

Morning Sleep Journal

Complete this each morning to see the impact on your daily sleep!

Today's Date: _____   Bedtime Last Night: _____

How well did you fall asleep?

___ Easily   ___ It took a while   ___ It was difficult

Describe what it was like falling asleep:

Did you wake up and struggle to fall back asleep?

___ Not at all   ___ Once or twice   ___ Multiple times

Describe your experience:

Wake-Up Time: _____   Total Hours of Sleep _____

How did you feel after waking up?

___ Refreshed   ___ Just okay   ___ Tired

Notes:

Low Blood Sugar (Hypoglycemia)

Because balanced blood sugar levels are crucial to your survival, when blood sugar levels drop too low, your body thinks you are in a state of emergency. It responds by releasing the stress hormones cortisol and adrenaline to help raise blood sugar back to normal levels. As you are now aware, cortisol is the antithesis of melatonin. In addition, these hormones can stimulate your nervous system, leading to increased alertness and difficulty falling asleep or staying asleep (another reason you could be jarred awake at 3:00 am.) Hypoglycemia can also cause symptoms such as night sweats, nightmares, and restless sleep.

Sleep Apnea and High Blood Sugar (hyperglycemia)

High blood sugar levels can contribute to the development of sleep apnea, a condition characterized by pauses in breathing during sleep. Sleep apnea can disrupt sleep and lead to daytime fatigue, as well as increase the risk of other health issues like high blood pressure and heart disease.

Insulin Resistance and Poor Sleep Quality

Insulin resistance, a common feature of type 2 diabetes and metabolic syndrome, can also affect sleep quality. Studies have shown that individuals with insulin resistance often experience poorer sleep quality, longer sleep onset times, and more nighttime awakenings. To maintain stable levels:

- Eat regular, balanced meals throughout the day, with a mix of protein, healthy fats, and complex carbohydrates.

- Aim for a mostly whole foods diet (made in nature) and limit processed foods (made in a factory).

- Avoid consuming large meals or sugary snacks close to bedtime, as this can lead to blood sugar fluctuations during the night.

- Engage in regular physical activity (early in the day), which can help improve insulin sensitivity and blood sugar regulation.

- Manage stress, as chronic stress can contribute to both blood sugar dysregulation and sleep issues.

- Talk to your healthcare provider about checking your blood sugar levels.

Addressing blood sugar imbalances and adopting a healthy lifestyle can improve sleep quality and overall well-being.

Evening Sleep Journal

Incorporate this journal into your evening wind-down routine.

Today's Date: _____

Write down the time/description for each item.

Caffeine	
Supplements	
Medications	
Exercise	
Evening Meal	
Snacks	
Beverages	
Alcohol	
Naps	

My Sleepiness Level Today (Low / Medium / High)

My Stress Level Today (Low / Medium / High)

Can you make any connections to activities that impacted sleep?

DAY 30

Hormone Havoc

From your first period through the valley of menopause, fluctuating hormones can have a significant impact on sleep quality in women. As you may know, one of the most common symptoms of sleep disruptors in this arena is the dreaded night sweats.

There's nothing like waking up in the middle of the night with soaking wet PJs and damp sheets. While I was going through menopause, my husband said it was like sleeping with a furnace. If you are dealing with night sweats due to fluctuating hormones, cooling off should be your first line of defense.

Go ahead with your Morning Sleep Journal, and then I will share all my best tips.

Morning Sleep Journal

Complete this each morning to see the impact on your daily sleep!

Today's Date: _____   Bedtime Last Night: _____

How well did you fall asleep?

___ Easily   ___ It took a while   ___ It was difficult

Describe what it was like falling asleep:

Did you wake up and struggle to fall back asleep?

___ Not at all   ___ Once or twice   ___ Multiple times

Describe your experience:

Wake-Up Time: _____   Total Hours of Sleep _____

How did you feel after waking up?

___ Refreshed   ___ Just okay   ___ Tired

Notes:

Tackling Night Sweats

Battling night sweats begins with temperature regulation. Ensuring your room is cool can make a significant difference. But sometimes, it's more about managing your internal thermostat than the room's:

Cool Down Before Bed

A lukewarm shower or bath can help lower your core temperature, prepping your body for sleep.

Opt for Breathable Bedding

Specialized sheets and pillowcases, often made from materials like bamboo or moisture-wicking fabrics, can keep you cool throughout the night.

Maximize Air Circulation

Use ceiling or oscillating fans to promote air movement. On cooler nights, crack open a window for some fresh, chilly air.

Dress Smartly

Choose lightweight, moisture-wicking sleepwear.

When Natural Means Are Not Enough

Sometimes, despite all efforts, those hormonal surges are just too powerful. If natural cooling methods aren't providing relief, consider consulting with a healthcare professional. They might recommend hormone therapies or natural supplements. You should also consult your doctor if you are on prescription medications to prevent an adverse interaction.

Black Cohosh

Historically used to relieve menopausal symptoms.

St. John's Wort

Often used for mood stabilization and can be beneficial for those dealing with mood swings during menopause.

Thiamine & Vitamin E

Both can support nerve function and reduce cramping during menstruation.

Magnesium & Omega-3 Fatty Acids

These are vital for various bodily functions, including hormone regulation. While hormonal shifts are an inevitable part of a woman's journey, remember that you're not alone in facing these challenges. With the right tools and information, you can find relief and get back to restful nights.

Evening Sleep Journal

Incorporate this journal into your evening wind-down routine.

Today's Date: _____

Write down the time/description for each item.

Caffeine	
Supplements	
Medications	
Exercise	
Evening Meal	
Snacks	
Beverages	
Alcohol	
Naps	

My Sleepiness Level Today (Low / Medium / High)

My Stress Level Today (Low / Medium / High)

Can you make any connections to activities that impacted sleep?

DAY 31

Dehydration and Nocturia

Another sneaky sleep stealer could be dehydration. Our bodies are water-loving machines that use the good ol' H2O for so many things – and when it comes to catching some quality zzz's, water plays a starring role too.

Think of it like this: when your body isn't getting enough water, it can dry up your mouth and throat, making you the star snorer of the house, or even set you up for a date with sleep apnea. Neither of these is particularly friendly to your sleep cycle. Oh, and those late-night leg cramps you've been blaming on over-exertion. Yep, dehydration could be the culprit behind those, too.

Before we get started, remember to fill out your Morning Sleep Journal for today.

Morning Sleep Journal

Complete this each morning to see the impact on your daily sleep!

Today's Date: _____   Bedtime Last Night: _____

How well did you fall asleep?

___ Easily   ____ It took a while   ____ It was difficult

Describe what it was like falling asleep:

Did you wake up and struggle to fall back asleep?

___ Not at all   ____ Once or twice   ____ Multiple times

Describe your experience:

Wake-Up Time: _____   Total Hours of Sleep _____

How did you feel after waking up?

___ Refreshed   ____ Just okay   ____ Tired

Notes:

Here's another shocker: dehydration can also play the villain in your body's melatonin production. When you're well-hydrated, your body can produce melatonin like a champ, which keeps your sleep-wake cycles in perfect harmony.

In addition, a parched body can trigger your heart to go a little wild at an increased rate and might even invite anxiety to the party, making it harder for you to fall asleep and stay asleep.

Now you see why hydration is a VIP guest in the world of good sleep hygiene, right? But remember, don't go chugging water right before bed, as midnight bathroom runs are not conducive to a good night's rest. So, just as you time your meals, check when you finish your water intake – a couple of hours before bedtime should do the trick.

Nocturia (Speaking of Water)

We've all been there—deep in the realms of dreamland when, suddenly, nature calls. That's 'nocturia' for you, a sleep-stealer that sends you trudging to the bathroom in the middle of the night. While it's a common occurrence as we age, consistent wake-up calls can seriously mess with your sleep quality.

Aside from that large glass of water before bedtime or certain medications, nocturia can also be a symptom of health issues such as diabetes or sleep disorders. If your midnight bathroom trips are becoming more frequent, it's definitely worth a chat with your healthcare provider.

Limit Fluid Intake: Avoid large amounts of fluids a couple of hours before bedtime.

Empty Bladder Fully: Ensure you've completely emptied your bladder before hitting the hay.

Munch on some Pumpkin Seeds: Also known as pepitas, these little gems are high in compounds that relax the bladder and keep it from contracting.

Spicy Lemonade: A quirky mix of cayenne pepper, lemon juice, and water believed by some to help. In fact, a study out of Thailand found that capsaicin in cayenne distracts overactive nerves in the bladder that tell your brain you have to go, increasing your bladder capacity by 63%.

Magnesium: Aiding muscle and nerve functions, these can calm bladder spasms, potentially reducing nighttime bathroom trips.

Leg Elevation: Standing on your feet all day can cause swollen legs and ankles. Gravity can pull the pooled fluids in swollen legs and ankles into your bladder. Try lifting those legs a while before you sleep to decrease the need for urination.

Remember, these tips aren't one-size-fits-all solutions. But they're worth exploring if you're on a quest for uninterrupted sleep. Always keep your healthcare provider informed about any changes or concerns you have. It might sound like we are saying it a lot - but that is because it is important!

Another thing that is important is for you to complete your Evening Sleep Journal for today.

Evening Sleep Journal

Incorporate this journal into your evening wind-down routine.

Today's Date: _____

Write down the time/description for each item.

Caffeine	
Supplements	
Medications	
Exercise	
Evening Meal	
Snacks	
Beverages	
Alcohol	
Naps	

My Sleepiness Level Today (Low / Medium / High)

My Stress Level Today (Low / Medium / High)

Can you make any connections to activities that impacted sleep?

DAY 32

Food Sensitivites

Did you ever think your dinner plate might hold some answers to your restless nights? We have already discussed the pitfalls of late, heavy dinners and blood sugar dysregulation. But those are not the only culprits. Food sensitivities can also be a hidden issue.

Today, we are going to examine the ways food might be affecting your sleep more closely. Right after you finish your Morning Sleep Journal.

Morning Sleep Journal

Complete this each morning to see the impact on your daily sleep!

Today's Date: _____   Bedtime Last Night: _____

How well did you fall asleep?

___ Easily   ___ It took a while   ___ It was difficult

Describe what it was like falling asleep:

Did you wake up and struggle to fall back asleep?

___ Not at all   ___ Once or twice   ___ Multiple times

Describe your experience:

Wake-Up Time: _____   Total Hours of Sleep _____

How did you feel after waking up?

___ Refreshed   ___ Just okay   ___ Tired

Notes:

Distinguishing Food Allergies from Sensitivities

Before we dive deep, let's clarify the difference between food allergies and sensitivities. Food allergies trigger an immediate immune response, which can be severe and even life-threatening, like the reaction some have to peanuts.

Food sensitivities, on the other hand, are sneakier. They might not produce an immediate reaction, and over time, you might just get used to the discomfort they cause without realizing the culprit. Common sensitivities include gluten, dairy, and eggs, but even foods considered healthy can be problematic for some. For instance, I have a sensitivity to certain vegetables.

You also should be aware of food additives that can trigger sensitivities in some individuals.

Monosodium Glutamate (MSG)

Often used as a flavor enhancer in many processed foods and in some restaurants. It's known to cause headaches or migraines in some people, among other symptoms.

Artificial Food Dyes

These can cause hyperactivity in children and allergic reactions in some individuals. Especially look for Red #40, Yellow #5 (Tartrazine), and Blue #1.

Sulfites

Found in dried fruits, wine, and some processed foods. They can trigger asthma attacks in those who are sulfite-sensitive.

Aspartame

A low-calorie artificial sweetener. Some reports suggest it might cause headaches, dizziness, and digestive symptoms for some people.

BHA and BHT

Butylated hydroxyanisole (BHA) and butylated hydroxytoluene (BHT) are preservatives used in many processed foods. They are known to cause allergic reactions and potentially other health concerns.

Nitrates and Nitrites

These are preservatives often found in processed meats. They can cause headaches and are linked to certain cancers.

Guar Gum

Used as a thickener in many processed foods, some people find they have digestive symptoms after consuming products with guar gum.

Carrageenan

Found in many dairy products and dairy alternatives, carrageenan can cause digestive distress for some individuals.

Polysorbate 80

An emulsifier often used in ice creams this can cause allergic reactions in some individuals.

Maltodextrin

Found in many processed foods, maltodextrin can cause spikes in blood sugar and might also affect gut bacteria.

When addressing sensitivities to these ingredients, it's important to read food labels thoroughly.

Detecting Food Sensitivities

There are a couple of approaches to identifying food sensitivities.

Food Sensitivity Testing

Such tests typically measure antibody levels in response to different foods. Depending on the test, they can pinpoint foods that your body might be reacting to subtly. Ask your healthcare provider about your options.

Histamine Intolerance and Sleep

Histamine, commonly known for its role in allergic reactions, also plays a part in regulating sleep-wake cycles. However, for those with histamine intolerance, an imbalance occurs when the body accumulates more histamine than it can efficiently break down. This intolerance can result from various factors, including gut health issues, certain medications, or consuming foods high in histamine.

Symptoms might include headaches, skin rashes, digestive problems, and, notably, sleep disturbances. Elevated histamine levels can lead to increased alertness, making it challenging to fall or stay asleep.

If you suspect histamine might impact your sleep, it's worth considering a low-histamine diet and consulting with a healthcare professional to devise an appropriate strategy to address the underlying causes.

The Coca Pulse Test

The Coca Pulse Test is a simple way you can try at home to see if specific foods are troubling your body, making it harder for you to sleep. Here is how to take the test:

Step One: Relax and take four deep breaths. You want to make sure your body is in a parasympathetic state (aka calm).

Step Two: Measure your resting pulse for one full minute (set a timer). The easiest place to find your pulse is on your wrist or carotid artery in your neck. Press lightly with your index and middle finger until you feel the blood pumping. Count the beats for 60 seconds. Write it down.

Step Three: Place a small piece of the suspect food under your tongue for 30 seconds, then discard it. Your brain's "alert center" (called the hypothalamus) talks to your body's control system, checking if this food is a "bad guy".

Step Four: Repeat step two and measure your pulse for 60 seconds. Write down the result. An increase of more than six beats per minute may indicate a sensitivity to that food.

Step Five: To be certain, consider eliminating the food from your diet for a few weeks and monitor if your sleep improves.

190

The Gut-Sleep Connection

Often, food sensitivities are intertwined with gut health issues like increased intestinal permeability, often referred to as 'leaky gut'. Addressing gut health can sometimes alleviate food sensitivities. If you suspect you have food sensitivities, it's crucial to consult with a healthcare practitioner who can guide you through a comprehensive gut healing protocol.

Remember, food is fuel, but the wrong kind can throw off more than just your digestion. It might be the missing link in your quest for better sleep.

Evening Sleep Journal

Incorporate this journal into your evening wind-down routine.

Today's Date: _____

Write down the time/description for each item.

Caffeine	
Supplements	
Medications	
Exercise	
Evening Meal	
Snacks	
Beverages	
Alcohol	
Naps	

My Sleepiness Level Today (Low / Medium / High)

My Stress Level Today (Low / Medium / High)

Can you make any connections to activities that impacted sleep?

DAY 33

Sleep Disorders

If you have been implementing the sleep strategies outlined in this book and are not seeing results, it might indicate a deeper issue. Sleep disorders can significantly impact your quality of life, and while some might require simple lifestyle changes, others might necessitate professional intervention.

Let's take a look at some of the most common sleep disorders after the Morning Sleep Journal.

Morning Sleep Journal

Complete this each morning to see the impact on your daily sleep!

Today's Date: _____   Bedtime Last Night: _____

How well did you fall asleep?

___ Easily   ____ It took a while   ____ It was difficult

Describe what it was like falling asleep:

Did you wake up and struggle to fall back asleep?

___ Not at all   ____ Once or twice   ____ Multiple times

Describe your experience:

Wake-Up Time: _____   Total Hours of Sleep _____

How did you feel after waking up?

___ Refreshed   ____ Just okay   ____ Tired

Notes:

Sleep Apnea

Sleep apnea is characterized by brief interruptions of breathing during sleep. The most common type is obstructive sleep apnea (OSA), where the throat muscles relax excessively.

Symptoms: Loud snoring, feeling tired even after a full night's sleep, sudden awakenings accompanied by choking or gasping, and difficulty staying asleep.

Professional Help: Diagnosis often involves a sleep study, and treatments can range from lifestyle changes and using a CPAP machine to surgery in severe cases.

Restless Legs Syndrome (RLS)

RLS causes an irresistible urge to move your legs, usually due to discomfort. It typically happens in the evenings, making it hard to fall asleep.

Symptoms: Unpleasant sensations in the legs are described as crawling, creeping, pulling, or itching, and a strong urge to move the legs to relieve the sensations.

Professional Help: Diagnosis is usually based on symptoms, and treatments can include lifestyle changes, physical therapy, and medications.

Narcolepsy

Narcolepsy is a chronic sleep disorder characterized by overwhelming daytime drowsiness and sudden attacks of sleep.

Symptoms: Excessive daytime sleepiness, sudden loss of muscle tone, sleep paralysis, and hallucinations.

Professional Help: Diagnosis might involve sleep studies, and treatment often includes medications and lifestyle changes.

Circadian Rhythm Sleep Disorders

Circadian Rhythm Sleep disorders involve a disruption in the timing of sleep, wakefulness, and other daily rhythms.

Symptoms: Difficulty falling asleep and staying asleep, trouble waking up in the morning, and daytime sleepiness.

Professional Help: Treatments often involve light therapy, behavioral strategies, and, in some cases, medications.

Parasomnias

Parasomnia refers to abnormal behaviors during sleep, such as sleepwalking or night terrors.

Symptoms: Sleepwalking, night terrors, nightmares, teeth grinding, or restless sleep.

Professional Help: Most parasomnias are diagnosed through patient history. Treatment focuses on safety, counseling, and, in some cases, medications.

If you suspect you might be dealing with one of these disorders, it's essential to consult with a sleep specialist. They can provide a clear diagnosis and guide you towards effective treatments, ensuring you get the restful sleep you deserve.

Evening Sleep Journal

Incorporate this journal into your evening wind-down routine.

Today's Date: _____

Write down the time/description for each item.

Caffeine	
Supplements	
Medications	
Exercise	
Evening Meal	
Snacks	
Beverages	
Alcohol	
Naps	

My Sleepiness Level Today (Low / Medium / High)

My Stress Level Today (Low / Medium / High)

Can you make any connections to activities that impacted sleep?

DAY 34

Solidifying Sleep Success and Planning Forward

Congratulations on completing your 5-week journey towards peaceful, restorative sleep! I hope you found it to be a worthwhile experience. Being your own sleep detective might feel overwhelming, but remember, you've now got the knowledge and the tools to unravel this mystery. You're equipped to understand your body's unique sleep needs and address potential issues that may be impacting your sleep quality.

We will wrap up with some final notes and then include the necessary resources to keep going!

But first, it is time for your Morning Sleep Journal.

Morning Sleep Journal

Complete this each morning to see the impact on your daily sleep!

Today's Date: _____   Bedtime Last Night: _____

How well did you fall asleep?

___ Easily   ___ It took a while   ___ It was difficult

Describe what it was like falling asleep:

Did you wake up and struggle to fall back asleep?

___ Not at all   ___ Once or twice   ___ Multiple times

Describe your experience:

Wake-Up Time: _____   Total Hours of Sleep _____

How did you feel after waking up?

___ Refreshed   ___ Just okay   ___ Tired

Notes:

Next Steps

If you've been exploring these areas and are still struggling to find the answers, don't be discouraged. Our bodies are complex systems, and it can take time to fully understand and adjust our habits to suit our individual needs. Stay patient and consistent in your quest for better sleep.

When to Get Help

If you suspect serious issues like sleep disorders, don't hesitate to consult with a healthcare professional. Sometimes, professional intervention is necessary to diagnose and treat conditions that are too complex for us to handle alone.

Keep Journaling

Keep your journal handy and continue logging your sleep patterns and changes. It will remain a valuable tool for identifying trends, assessing the effectiveness of changes, and revealing areas still needing attention.

And who knows? With the insights you've gained, you might just become the go-to sleep expert in your circle, guiding others on their own path to better sleep. Now, wouldn't that be a dream come true?

Remember, the journey to better sleep is not a sprint but a marathon. Some nights will be easier than others, and that's okay. You've started on the path, and every step you take brings you closer to the ultimate goal - waking up refreshed and revitalized, ready to embrace the new day.

Keep persevering, keep learning, and most importantly, keep sleeping. The puzzle of perfect sleep may not be solved overnight, but with patience and persistence, you'll continue making strides toward the peaceful slumber you deserve.

Action Item: Reflection

Over the past five weeks, you've diligently gathered knowledge and made proactive strides to enhance your sleep. Now, let's take a moment to reflect on your impressive progress.

Taking this time will ensure that you can continue the positive habits you have started for years to come.

Retake Your Sleep Assessment

Now that we've neared the end of the program, it's time to retake your sleep assessment. Note any changes or improvements from when you first began. Take the time to reflect on these changes and how they have impacted your overall well-being.

Sleep Journal Review

Look back over your sleep journal entries from the last few weeks. Look for patterns and connections between your daily activities, stress management techniques, and your sleep quality. This process of reflection can help you identify what's working well and what may still need adjustment.

Troubleshooting Checklist

If you find yourself still struggling with falling asleep or waking in the night, consult the troubleshooting checklist to pinpoint potential areas of concern. This list is designed to help you navigate and address the most common sleep disruptors based on the practices and insights covered in this book.

Reflections Journal

Complete the Reflections Document. Ask yourself: What have you learned about yourself and your sleep habits throughout this program? Have certain strategies or changes had a significant impact on your sleep? Which habits do you plan on keeping long-term?

Plan Your Sleep Journey Forward

Based on your experiences and learnings from the program, what else are you going to experiment with? Are there any strategies or techniques you haven't tried yet, but are willing to incorporate into your routine?

Celebrate Your Achievements

Last, but certainly not least, take a moment to celebrate your achievements! Whether you've made significant strides in improving your sleep or grown in self-awareness and understanding, every step is progress. Acknowledge the commitment and effort you've put into this journey and celebrate your progress, whether big or small.

Remember, the journey to better sleep doesn't end here. It's an ongoing process of learning and adjustment. This program has given you the tools and knowledge to continue this path independently. As you move forward, keep experimenting, adjusting, and fine-tuning your strategies for better sleep. You've got this!

Evening Sleep Journal

Incorporate this journal into your evening wind-down routine.

Today's Date: _____

Write down the time/description for each item.

Caffeine	
Supplements	
Medications	
Exercise	
Evening Meal	
Snacks	
Beverages	
Alcohol	
Naps	

My Sleepiness Level Today (Low / Medium / High)

My Stress Level Today (Low / Medium / High)

Can you make any connections to activities that impacted sleep?

NOW WHAT?

Thank you for joining me on this journey with 'RELAX, SLEEP, THRIVE!' I'm thrilled to have shared these insights with you, and I'm hopeful that you're already experiencing the bliss of peaceful, restorative sleep. But our time together does not have to end here. There's so much more I would like to share with you to enhance your sleep further.

Unlock Your Sleep Toolbox

Visit relaxsleepthrive.com and download your own Sleep Toolbox guide.

It's packed with links to my recommendations for sleep-enhancing products. You will also have access to extra journal pages and checklists, designed to deepen your understanding of your sleep patterns and help maintain your progress.

Stay Connected for More Tips and Updates: Follow me on Instagram @amanda.chocko for a regular dose of sleep wisdom, lifestyle tips, and updates on upcoming programs and events.

I'm excited to continue this journey with you!

Sleep well and dream big,

Amanda

RESOURCES

Everything You Need for Long-Term Success

Included in the Resources section you will find copies of all the tools you have come to rely on, as well as some new checklists and materials.

Refer to these and use them whenever you need to.

Best wishes and you continue your sleep journey!

Sweet dreams!

Sleep Assessment

This sleep assessment reveals the extent of your sleep problems.
Rate each symptom according to the scale below.

Point Scale:

(0) never (1) 1-2 days/week (2) 3- 4 days/week (3) 5-7 days/week

_____ I need alcohol or medications to relax before bed.

_____ I have trouble falling asleep

_____ I cannot fall asleep because I am worrying about things

_____ I wake up more than once during the night

_____ I toss and turn at night

_____ I wake up and need to go to the bathroom

_____ I wake up before my alarm and cannot fall back asleep

_____ I have trouble waking up

_____ I need caffeine in the morning to get me going

_____ I have trouble concentrating during the day

_____ I have night sweats

_____ I wake up suddenly with a strong sense of anxiety

_____ I have difficulty falling asleep because of chronic pain

_____ I am sleepy during the day

_____ I find myself irritable or unable to tolerate normal stress

_____ I often have a hard time remembering things

_____ I doze off during the day while working and/or driving

_____ I often feel like I am in a daze or brain fog

_____ **Total Score**

Morning Sleep Journal

Complete this each morning to see the impact on your daily sleep!

Today's Date: _____   Bedtime Last Night: _____

How well did you fall asleep?

___ Easily   ____ It took a while   ____ It was difficult

Describe what it was like falling asleep:

Did you wake up and struggle to fall back asleep?

___ Not at all   ____ Once or twice   ____ Multiple times

Wake-Up Time: _____   Total Hours of Sleep _____

How did you feel after waking up?

___ Refreshed   ____ Just okay   ____ Tired

Notes:

Describe your experience:

Evening Sleep Journal

Incorporate this journal into your evening wind-down routine.

Today's Date: _____

Write down the time/description for each item.

Caffeine	
Supplements	
Medications	
Exercise	
Evening Meal	
Snacks	
Beverages	
Alcohol	
Naps	

My Sleepiness Level Today (Low / Medium / High)

My Stress Level Today (Low / Medium / High)

Can you make any connections to activities that impacted sleep?

Reframing Worksheet

Use this tool whenever you need help managing stressful thoughts.

Today's Date: _____

Step One: Identify the Negative Thought

What is the negative or recurring thought? What event triggered this thought?

Step Two: Challenge the Thought

Is there any evidence that this is true? Is there evidence that this thought may be false?

Step Three: Reframe the Thought

What is the worst thing that could happen if this thought came true? What is the most likely thing to happen? Is there anything I can do about this? Is there another way to look at this?

Step Four: New Thought

Troubleshooting Checklist #1

Trouble Falling Asleep

Today's Date: _____

☐ **Consistent Sleep Schedule**
Ensure that you're sticking to your routine. Remember the importance of regular sleep and wake times to anchor your body's internal clock.

☐ **Wind Down Routine**
Reflect on the winding down practices you've adopted. Are you giving your mind and body the cues they need to prepare for sleep?

☐ **Sleep Sanctuary**
Ensure your sleeping environment is conducive to rest. Is it dark, cool, and quiet? Have you eliminated electronic distractions and check that your mattress and pillows are comfortable?

☐ **Light Exposure**
Limit exposure to screens and bright lights in the evening. Remember the importance of natural light exposure during the day to regulate your circadian rhythm.

☐ **Stress Management Techniques**
Draw from the arsenal of relaxation exercises in the book. This could be deep breathing, progressive muscle relaxation, or designated worry time.

☐ **Timing of Daily Activities**
Pay close attention to the timing of caffeine and alcohol consumption and the size and timing of your meals. These can all play a role in your sleep quality.

Troubleshooting Checklist #2

Waking in the Night

Today's Date: _____

☐ **Nocturia**
Are frequent bathroom trips disturbing your sleep? Assess your fluid intake before bed.

☐ **Alcohol Consumption**
While alcohol might help you fall asleep, it can disturb your sleep cycle later in the night. Monitor and limit your intake, especially close to bedtime.

☐ **Food Sensitivities**
Recall our discussions on food sensitivities. These could be subtly affecting your sleep. Consider any recent dietary changes and their potential impacts.

☐ **Blood Sugar**
A significant drop in blood sugar can wake you up. Make sure your last meal or snack before bed isn't too high in sugars.

☐ **Pain Management**
If physical discomfort is a factor, investigate potential causes and remedies. This might mean revisiting your mattress choice or seeking medical advice.

☐ **Tips for Waking in the Night**
If you find yourself consistently waking up and unable to return to sleep, remember not to lie in bed awake for too long. After 10-15 minutes, get up and engage in a calming activity until you feel sleepy again.

Reflections Journal
Use this as a prompt to keep moving forward.

Today's Date: _____

What have you learned about yourself and your sleep habits through this program?

Have certain strategies or changes had a significant impact on your sleep quality and/or quantity?

What habits do. youplan on keeping long-term?

According to your Sleep Assessment, which areas still need work?

Based on your experiences and learnings from the program, what else are you going to experiment with?

Are there any strategies or techniques you haven't tried yet, but are willing to incorporate into your routine?

REFERENCES

Week 2: The Sleep Scholar

Cognitive impairment in individuals with insomnia: clinical significance and correlates (pubmed)
Fortier-Brochu E, Morin CM. Cognitive impairment in individuals with insomnia: clinical significance and correlates. Sleep. 2014 Nov 1;37(11):1787-98. doi: 10.5665/sleep.4172. PMID: 25364074; PMCID: PMC4196062.

Sleep and emotions: a focus on insomnia
Baglioni C, Spiegelhalder K, Lombardo C, Riemann D. Sleep and emotions: a focus on insomnia. Sleep Med Rev. 2010 Aug;14(4):227-38. doi: 10.1016/j.smrv.2009.10.007. Epub 2010 Feb 6. PMID: 20137989.

The association of insomnia disorder characterised by objective short sleep duration with hypertension, diabetes and body mass index: A systematic review and meta-analysis
Johnson KA, Gordon CJ, Chapman JL, Hoyos CM, Marshall NS, Miller CB, Grunstein RR. The association of insomnia disorder characterised by objective short sleep duration with hypertension, diabetes and body mass index: A systematic review and meta-analysis. Sleep Med Rev. 2021 Oct;59:101456. doi: 10.1016/j.smrv.2021.101456. Epub 2021 Jan 23. PMID: 33640704. 16. PMID: 35575450; PMCID: PMC9541543.

REFERENCES

Comorbid insomnia and sleep apnoea is associated with all-cause mortality
Lechat B, Appleton S, Melaku YA, Hansen K, McEvoy RD, Adams R, Catcheside P, Lack L, Eckert DJ, Sweetman A. Comorbid insomnia and sleep apnoea is associated with all-cause mortality. Eur Respir J. 2022 Jul 13;60(1):2101958. doi: 10.1183/13993003.01958-2021. PMID: 34857613.

The Neurobiology of Circadian Rhythms
Sollars PJ, Pickard GE. The Neurobiology of Circadian Rhythms. Psychiatr Clin North Am. 2015 Dec;38(4):645-65. doi: 10.1016/j.psc.2015.07.003. Epub 2015 Sep 5. PMID: 26600101; PMCID: PMC4660252.

Adenosine, caffeine, and sleep-wake regulation: state of the science and perspectives
Reichert CF, Deboer T, Landolt HP. Adenosine, caffeine, and sleep-wake regulation: state of the science and perspectives. J Sleep Res. 2022 Aug;31(4):e13597. doi: 10.1111/jsr.13597. Epub 2022 May 16. PMID: 35575450; PMCID: PMC9541543.

Physiology, Sleep Stages
Authors Aakash K. Patel1; Vamsi Reddy2; Karlie R. Shumway3; John F. Araujo4. National Library of Medicine

REFERENCES

Week 3: The Sleep Detective

Association between light at night, melatonin secretion, sleep deprivation, and the internal clock: Health impacts and mechanisms of circadian disruption
Touitou Y, Reinberg A, Touitou D. Association between light at night, melatonin secretion, sleep deprivation, and the internal clock: Health impacts and mechanisms of circadian disruption. Life Sci. 2017 Mar 15;173:94-106. doi: 10.1016/j.lfs.2017.02.008. Epub 2017 Feb 16. PMID: 28214594.

How Bad Is It Really to Work Out Right Before Bed?
Livestrong.Com Author-Leah Groth,

Circadian rhythms and meal timing: impact on energy balance and body weight
Boege HL, Bhatti MZ, St-Onge MP. Circadian rhythms and meal timing: impact on energy balance and body weight. Curr Opin Biotechnol. 2021 Aug;70:1-6. doi: 10.1016/j.copbio.2020.08.009. Epub 2020 Sep 29. PMID: 32998085; PMCID: PMC7997809.

7 Really Surprising Vitamins That Keep You Awake at Night
Written by Louise Carter Sleep Bubble

Alcohol and sleep I: effects on normal sleep
Ebrahim IO, Shapiro CM, Williams AJ, Fenwick PB. Alcohol and sleep I: effects on normal sleep. Alcohol Clin Exp Res. 2013 Apr;37(4):539-49. doi: 10.1111/acer.12006. Epub 2013 Jan 24. PMID: 23347102.

10 Common Medications That Can Affect Sleep By Ashley Garling, Pharm.D, AARP
Published April 08, 2013 / Updated June 30, 2023

REFERENCES

Week 4: Mastering Mind Management

The impact of stress on sleep: Pathogenic sleep reactivity as a vulnerability to insomnia and circadian disorders
Kalmbach DA, Anderson JR, Drake CL. The impact of stress on sleep: Pathogenic sleep reactivity as a vulnerability to insomnia and circadian disorders. J Sleep Res. 2018 Dec;27(6):e12710. doi: 10.1111/jsr.12710. Epub 2018 May 24. PMID: 29797753; PMCID: PMC7045300.

Cognitive Restructuring Techniques for Reframing Thoughts 12 Feb 2018
by Courtney E. Ackerman, MA. Scientifically reviewed by Gabriella Lancia, Ph.D. PositivePsychology.com

Brief structured respiration practices enhance mood and reduce physiological arousal
Balban MY, Neri E, Kogon MM, Weed L, Nouriani B, Jo B, Holl G, Zeitzer JM, Spiegel D, Huberman AD. Brief structured respiration practices enhance mood and reduce physiological arousal. Cell Rep Med. 2023 Jan 17;4(1):100895. doi: 10.1016/j.xcrm.2022.100895. Epub 2023 Jan 10. PMID: 36630953; PMCID: PMC9873947.

The effect of mindfulness meditation on sleep quality: a systematic review and meta-analysis of randomized controlled trials
Rusch HL, Rosario M, Levison LM, Olivera A, Livingston WS, Wu T, Gill JM. The effect of mindfulness meditation on sleep quality: a systematic review and meta-analysis of randomized controlled trials. Ann N Y Acad Sci. 2019 Jun;1445(1):5-16. doi: 10.1111/nyas.13996. Epub 2018 Dec 21. PMID: 30575050; PMCID: PMC6557693.

REFERENCES

Week 5: The Sleep Hacker

Noise as a sleep aid: A systematic review
Riedy SM, Smith MG, Rocha S, Basner M. Noise as a sleep aid: A systematic review. Sleep Med Rev. 2021 Feb;55:101385. doi: 10.1016/j.smrv.2020.101385. Epub 2020 Sep 9. PMID: 33007706.

Towards Improving Sleep Quality Using Automatic Sleep Stage Classification and Binaural Beats
Munoz JP, Rivera LA. Towards Improving Sleep Quality Using Automatic Sleep Stage Classification and Binaural Beats. Annu Int Conf IEEE Eng Med Biol Soc. 2020 Jul;2020:4982-4985. doi: 10.1109/EMBC44109.2020.9176385. PMID: 33019105.

Wearing blue light-blocking glasses in the evening advances circadian rhythms in the patients with delayed sleep phase disorder: An open-label trial
Esaki Y, Kitajima T, Ito Y, Koike S, Nakao Y, Tsuchiya A, Hirose M, Iwata N. Wearing blue light-blocking glasses in the evening advances circadian rhythms in the patients with delayed sleep phase disorder: An open-label trial. Chronobiol Int. 2016;33(8):1037-44. doi: 10.1080/07420528.2016.1194289. Epub 2016 Jun 20. PMID: 27322730.

REFERENCES

The effectiveness of weighted blankets on sleep and everyday activities - A retrospective follow-up study of children and adults with attention deficit hyperactivity disorder and/or autism spectrum disorder
Bolic Baric V, Skuthälla S, Pettersson M, Gustafsson PA, Kjellberg A. The effectiveness of weighted blankets on sleep and everyday activities - A retrospective follow-up study of children and adults with attention deficit hyperactivity disorder and/or autism spectrum disorder. Scand J Occup Ther. 2021 Jun 29:1-11. doi: 10.1080/11038128.2021.1939414. Epub ahead of print. PMID: 34184958.

Effects of aromatherapy on sleep quality and anxiety of patients
Karadag E, Samancioglu S, Ozden D, Bakir E. Effects of aromatherapy on sleep quality and anxiety of patients. Nurs Crit Care. 2017 Mar;22(2):105-112. doi: 10.1111/nicc.12198. Epub 2015 Jul 27. PMID: 26211735.

Effect of melatonin supplementation on sleep quality: a systematic review and meta-analysis of randomized controlled trials
Fatemeh G, Sajjad M, Niloufar R, Neda S, Leila S, Khadijeh M. Effect of melatonin supplementation on sleep quality: a systematic review and meta-analysis of randomized controlled trials. J Neurol. 2022 Jan;269(1):205-216. doi: 10.1007/s00415-020-10381-w. Epub 2021 Jan 8. PMID: 33417003.

Valerian Root in Treating Sleep Problems and Associated Disorders-A Systematic Review and Meta-Analysis
Shinjyo N, Waddell G, Green J. Valerian Root in Treating Sleep Problems and Associated Disorders-A Systematic Review and Meta-Analysis. J Evid Based Integr Med. 2020 Jan-Dec;25:2515690X20967323. doi: 10.1177/2515690X20967323. PMID: 33086877; PMCID: PMC7585905.

REFERENCES

Cannabis, Cannabinoids, and Sleep: a Review of the Literature Babson KA, Sottile J, Morabito D. Cannabis, Cannabinoids, and Sleep: a Review of the Literature. Curr Psychiatry Rep. 2017 Apr;19(4):23. doi: 10.1007/s11920-017-0775-9. PMID: 28349316.

Adaptogenic and Anxiolytic Effects of Ashwagandha Root Extract in Healthy Adults: A Double-blind, Randomized, Placebo-controlled Clinical Study Salve J, Pate S, Debnath K, Langade D. Adaptogenic and Anxiolytic Effects of Ashwagandha Root Extract in Healthy Adults: A Double-blind, Randomized, Placebo-controlled Clinical Study. Cureus. 2019 Dec 25;11(12):e6466. doi: 10.7759/cureus.6466. PMID: 32021735; PMCID: PMC6979308.

REFERENCES

Week 6: The Sleep Strategist

Hydration and Sleep
Updated February 2, 2023 Dr. Abhinav Singh. Sleep Foundation

Insomnia and menopause: a narrative review on mechanisms and treatments
Proserpio P, Marra S, Campana C, Agostoni EC, Palagini L, Nobili L, Nappi RE. Insomnia and menopause: a narrative review on mechanisms and treatments. Climacteric. 2020 Dec;23(6):539-549. doi: 10.1080/13697137.2020.1799973. Epub 2020 Sep 3. PMID: 32880197.

Nocturia × disturbed sleep: a review
Furtado D, Hachul H, Andersen ML, Castro RA, Girão MB, Tufik S. Nocturia × disturbed sleep: a review. Int Urogynecol J. 2012 Mar;23(3):255-67. doi: 10.1007/s00192-011-1525-x. Epub 2011 Aug 17. PMID: 22052440.

The Epidemiology of Sleep and Diabetes
Ogilvie RP, Patel SR. The Epidemiology of Sleep and Diabetes. Curr Diab Rep. 2018 Aug 17;18(10):82. doi: 10.1007/s11892-018-1055-8. PMID: 30120578; PMCID: PMC6437687.

REFERENCES

Week 6: The Sleep Strategist

Hydration and Sleep
Updated February 2, 2023 Dr. Abhinav Singh. Sleep Foundation

Insomnia and menopause: a narrative review on mechanisms and treatments
Proserpio P, Marra S, Campana C, Agostoni EC, Palagini L, Nobili L, Nappi RE. Insomnia and menopause: a narrative review on mechanisms and treatments. Climacteric. 2020 Dec;23(6):539-549. doi: 10.1080/13697137.2020.1799973. Epub 2020 Sep 3. PMID: 32880197.

Nocturia × disturbed sleep: a review
Furtado D, Hachul H, Andersen ML, Castro RA, Girão MB, Tufik S. Nocturia × disturbed sleep: a review. Int Urogynecol J. 2012 Mar;23(3):255-67. doi: 10.1007/s00192-011-1525-x. Epub 2011 Aug 17. PMID: 22052440.

The Epidemiology of Sleep and Diabetes
Ogilvie RP, Patel SR. The Epidemiology of Sleep and Diabetes. Curr Diab Rep. 2018 Aug 17;18(10):82. doi: 10.1007/s11892-018-1055-8. PMID: 30120578; PMCID: PMC6437687.

www.ingramcontent.com/pod-product-compliance
Lightning Source LLC
Chambersburg PA
CBHW071156130626

46553CB00004B/1684